Ankle Arthroscopy

PATHOLOGY AND SURGICAL TECHNIQUES

Ankle Arthroscopy

PATHOLOGY AND SURGICAL TECHNIQUES

James F Guhl MD

SLACK Incorporated, 6900 Grove Road, Thorofare, New Jersey 08086

Copyright © 1988 by SLACK Incorporated

All rights reserved. No part of this book may be reproduced, stored in a retrieval system or transmitted in any form or by any means, electronic, mechanical, photocopying, recording or otherwise, without written permission from the publisher, except for brief quotations embodied in critical articles and reviews.

Printed in the United States of America

Library of Congress Catalog Card Number: 87-62917

ISBN: 0-943432-62-6

Published by: SLACK Incorporated
6900 Grove Rd.
Thorofare, NJ 08086

Last digit is print number: 10   9   8   7   6   5   4   3   2   1

Contents

	Preface	ix
	Contributors	xi
Chapter 1	**History and Development** *James F. Guhl, M.D.*	1
Chapter 2	**Gross Anatomy of the Ankle Joint** *Michael Harty, M.D., M.Ch., F.R.C.S (Eng)*	7
Chapter 3	**Arthroscopic Anatomy** *Dinesh Patel, M.D.* *James F. Guhl, M.D.*	13
Chapter 4	**Radiological Techniques** *C.F. Carrera, M.D.* *James F. Guhl, M.D.*	25
Chapter 5	**Instrumentation in Arthroscopic Surgery of the Ankle** *J. Serge Parisien, M.D.*	37
Chapter 6	**Portals and Techniques** *James F. Guhl, M.D.*	49
Chapter 7	**Indications and Contraindications** *George J. Schonholtz, M.D.*	63
Chapter 8	**Differential Diagnosis of Ankle Problems** *William G. Hamilton, M.D.*	69
Chapter 9	**Soft Tissue (Synovial) Pathology** *James F. Guhl, M.D.*	79
Chapter 10	**Osteochondritis Dissecans** *James F. Guhl, M.D.*	95
Chapter 11	**Other Chondral and Osteochondral Lesions** *James F. Guhl, M.D.*	107

Chapter 12	**Arthroscopic Tibiotalar Arthrodesis** *Craig D. Morgan, M.D.*	**119**
Chapter 13	**Stapling Repair for Chronic Lateral Ankle Instability** *Richard B. Hawkins, M.D.*	**123**
Chapter 14	**Arthroscopy of the Subtalar Joint (Posterior Subtalar Joint)** *J. Serge Parisien, M.D.*	**133**
Chapter 15	**Postoperative Care and Physical Therapy** *Harvey S. Kohn, M.D.* *Gary N. Guten, M.D.*	**143**
Chapter 16	**Complications** *James F. Guhl, M.D.*	**147**
Chapter 17	**Analysis and Conclusion** *James F. Guhl, M.D.*	**153**
	Index	**159**

Acknowledgments

The contributors to this book were chosen because of individual expertise in their particular fields, for which I am deeply indebted.

I am particularly grateful to the late Dr. Richard O'Connor, Drs. Lanny Johnson, Hiroshi Ikeuchi, Bob Jackson, John Joyce, Ward Casscells, and others. It is only because of the interest inspired in me by these men that I gained the insight and knowledge to hope to recognize these areas of concern and seek the answers.

My sincere thanks also is extended to Drs. Dean Furry, William Smith, Cliff Peterson, Joseph Manago, and Jeff Butler for their kind assistance in reviewing portions of this manuscript. I am also grateful to Drs. Richard Ferkel, Dennis Kasamian, Bert Mandelbaum, and Mark Meyerson for contributing their valuable illustrations.

Special thanks to David Strickland for his art work in accurately depicting the details in the medical illustrations.

This book would not have been written without the loyal support of my office staff: Barbara Fischer, Beth Ewens, and Joan Wehrman.

Finally, this book is dedicated to my long-suffering wife, Jane and my family: Steve and his wife Lori, Ann and her husband Dave, Tim, Tom, Mary, David, and my grandchildren Aileen, Benjamin, and Jessica.

Preface

The techniques in this monograph were developed from past experiences where dissatisfaction and frustration in performing ankle arthroscopy were encountered. Between 1975 and 1985 many different methods of arthroscopic treatment of the ankle joint were developed and taught in various courses in arthroscopic surgery. In early 1980, arthroscopy of the shoulder joint was gradually mastered and some work was done in the other joints, including the ankle. In the latter, in particular, there are great limitations, primarily caused by tight ligaments resulting in considerable space limitations. In addition, there is the anatomic curved configuration of the talocrural articulation, the anatomical structures blocking access to the joint (including the malleoli), and the neurovascular structures which impose additional problems.

There is further difficulty in triangulation, especially when employing the posterolateral approach, because of positional problems. For these reasons, diagnostic and operative arthroscopy was limited primarily to procedures which could be done in and around the anterior third of the joint with the patient supine and the extremity extended. The posterior compartment could be entered with adequate distention, but also with great difficulty. There was even a greater challenge encountered in triangulating and performing any meaningful operative procedures. Therefore, significant lesions in the mid- and posterior joint were often left undiagnosed and untreated. Manual distraction by the strongest assistant was not sufficient and this also could not be adequately maintained.

Other positions, such as the lateral decubitus position (with the patient supine, the thigh in a leg holder, the knee flexed, and the ankle dependent), were tried and found unsatisfactory.

With this experience and these problems in mind, various solutions were developed. These include the use of the mechanical distractor, transmalleolar approaches, improved instrumentation, and an ankle holder allowing easier use of the posterior approaches. Upon employing these techniques, a surprising amount previously unknown or unappreciated pathology was encountered and treated.

Certainly, the ankle will not approach the knee and perhaps the shoulder in the need for diagnostic and surgical procedures done arthroscopically. Nevertheless, the author expects that these newer techniques will open the door to further advances in arthroscopy of that joint.

Before recognizing these problems and arriving at logical conclusions, the author felt it necessary to have gained a considerable amount of experience in ankle arthroscopy. Also, extensive experience in the field of arthroscopic surgery appeared necessary in retrospect. The author therefore believes that, in order to appreciate these problems and develop some solutions, expertise, knowledge, and background gained in working with and learning from some of the giants in this field of endeavor was necessary.

It seems fitting at this point to compare the acquisition of knowledge portrayed in this text to a comment once mentioned to me by Dr. Richard O'Connor in respect to the comparison of a first series of 69 cases fraught with frustration to a second series where the problems were successfully solved by the introduction of the new techniques described throughout this book: "Good surgical technique is gained from experience — experience is acquired from poor surgery."

Contributors

James F. Guhl, M.D.
Department of Orthopaedics
St. Francis Hospital
Milwaukee, Wisconsin
Assistant Clinical Professor
Department of Orthopaedic Surgery
Medical College of Wisconsin
Past President, Arthroscopy Association
of North America
Secretary, International Arthroscopy Association
Member, Board of Trustees
Arthroscopy Journal

Guillermo Carrera, M.D.
Professor of Radiology
Department of Radiology
Chief of Diagnostic Radiology
Milwaukee County Medical Complex
Milwaukee, Wisconsin

Gary N. Guten, M.D.
Associate Clinical Professor
Medical College of Wisconsin
Milwaukee, Wisconsin

William Hamilton, M.D.
Assistant Clinical Professor
of Orthopaedic Surgery
Columbia University
College of Physicians and Surgeons
St. Luke's and Roosevelt Hospital
Orthopedist for the New York City Ballet,
the American Ballet Theatre,
and the School of the American Ballet
New York, New York

Michael Harty, M.D.
Professor Emeritus of Anatomy
University of Pennsylvania
Philadelphia, Pennsylvania

Richard Hawkins, M.D.
Orthopedic Surgeon
John Fitch Orthopaedics Associates
Fitchburg, Massachusetts

Harvey S. Kohn, M.D.
Clinical Instructor
Medical College of Wisconsin
Milwaukee, Wisconsin

Craig Morgan, M.D.
Medical Center of Delaware
St. Francis Hospital
Alfred I. DuPont Institute
University of Delaware
Wilmington, Delaware

Serge Parisien, M.D.
Chief of Arthroscopic Surgery Service
Hospital for Joint Disease
Orthopaedic Institute
New York, New York

Dinesh Patel, M.D.
Chief of Arthroscopic Surgery Unit
Massachusetts General Hospital
Harvard Medical School
Boston, Massachusetts

George Schonholtz, M.D.
President, Arthroscopy
Association of North America
Assistant Clinical Professor
of Orthopaedics
George Washington University
Civilian Consultant,
Walter Reed Army Medical Center
Silver Spring, Maryland

CHAPTER 1

HISTORY AND DEVELOPMENT

James F. Guhl, M.D.

Between 1974 and 1986 the author performed approximately 4,000 arthroscopic procedures. One hundred and thirty-one were cases of the ankle joint, 58 of these by the new technique that is the subject of this text.

Initially there was a considerable degree of dissatisfaction with the use of the small diameter arthroscope to see into a restricted ankle joint. The configuration of this articulation made the placement of the arthroscope and its advancement quite difficult. The prospect of performing diagnostic procedures, much less any surgical exercises, seemed rather dim and discouraging for the next several years. Interest therefore waned.

In 1977 the author had the opportunity of seeing Johnson[3] perform arthroscopy of the ankle (Figure 1-1). In April of 1977, in Nice, France, Ikeuchi presented a paper on ankle arthroscopy during a course in orthopedic surgery sponsored by the University of Pennsylvania. His presentation stimulated the interest of the author. It was obvious that Ikeuchi was able to

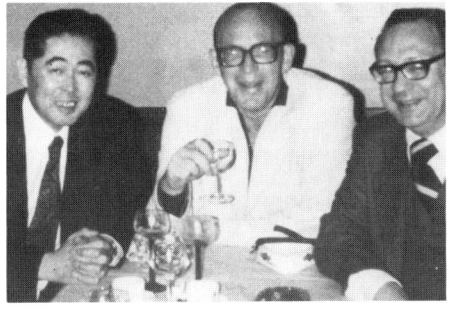

Figure 1-1. Dr. Hiroshi Ikeuchi, shown at the left, was the first orthopedic surgeon to perform operative arthroscopy and later develop ankle arthroscopy. The late Dr. Richard O'Connor, a pioneer in arthroscopic surgery in this country, is also shown as well as the author.

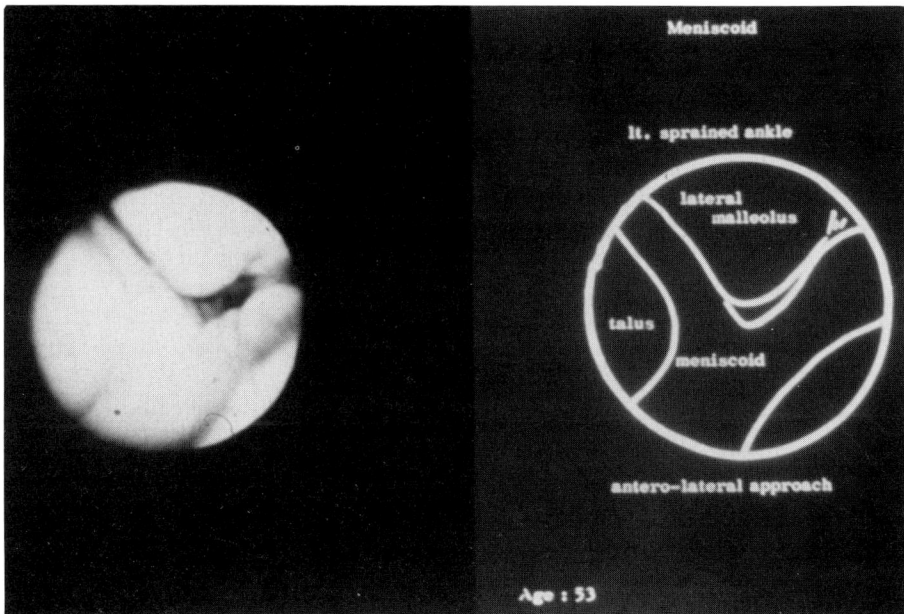

Figure 1-2. This illustration shows the meniscoid of the ankle, also illustrated in the diagram to the right.

see and diagnose cases of chronic synovitis, obtain biopsies, and show examples of chondral fractures and other lesions (Figures 1-2 through 1-5) with the Watanabe #25 arthroscope. He also described the meniscoid of the ankle as a definite soft tissue pathological entity that was responsible for chronic, longstanding, disabling pain. The development of this pathological structure followed certain types of inversion and supination injuries. These injuries, although not common, were also known to occur fairly often in athletes. Ikeuchi referred to Wolin's[2] original description of this entity and its pathological significance in *Surgery, Gynecology and Obstetrics*, 1952. At the same time, after observing Johnson's technique, the author was further encouraged by his use of the needlescope (Figures 1-6 and 1-7) for ankle arthroscopy. The latter technique incorporated the use of the halo, a fiber optic bundle surrounding the initial lens system of the needlescope. The halo was used to augment the amount of light for a more accurate view of the interior of the ankle and its lesions.

There was still, however, significant limitation in the ability to see and evaluate the entire structure and to triangulate accurately. This caused difficulty in properly placing and utilizing instruments, as well as in satisfactorily positioning the patient. The prone, supine, and lateral decubitus positions, or a combination of them, were employed. Placing the leg over the end of the table and using a knee holder was also tried. Certain lesions could not be adequately or safely reached by these methods for example drilling and debriding osteochondritis diseases of the talus, or treatment of articular cartilage and synoval lesions. Scuffing was a significant problem. Lesions of the anterior compartment, such as loose bodies and osteophytes, became relatively easy to see. Pathology of the posterior compartment and the mid-

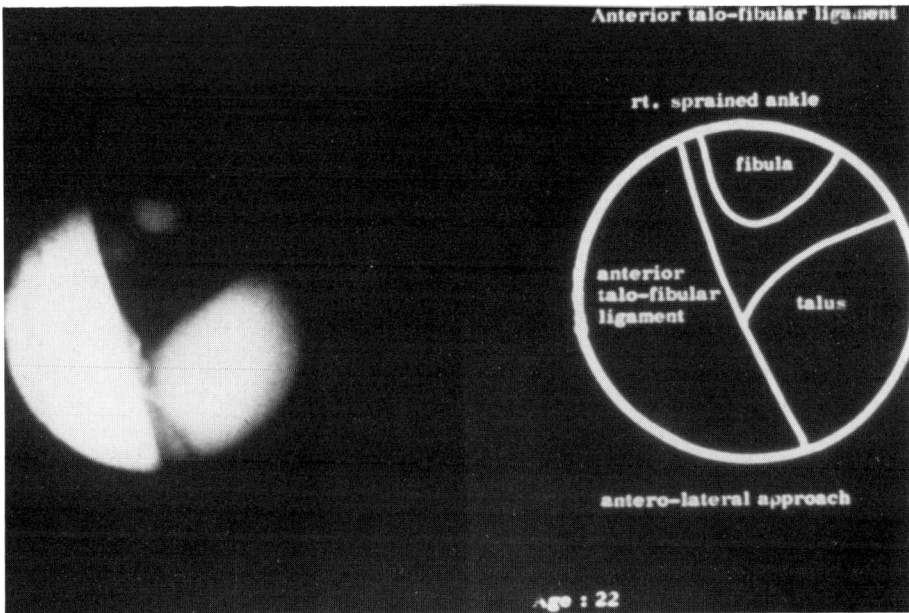

Figure 1-3. This picture shows the anterior talofibular ligament, illustrated in the diagram on the right.

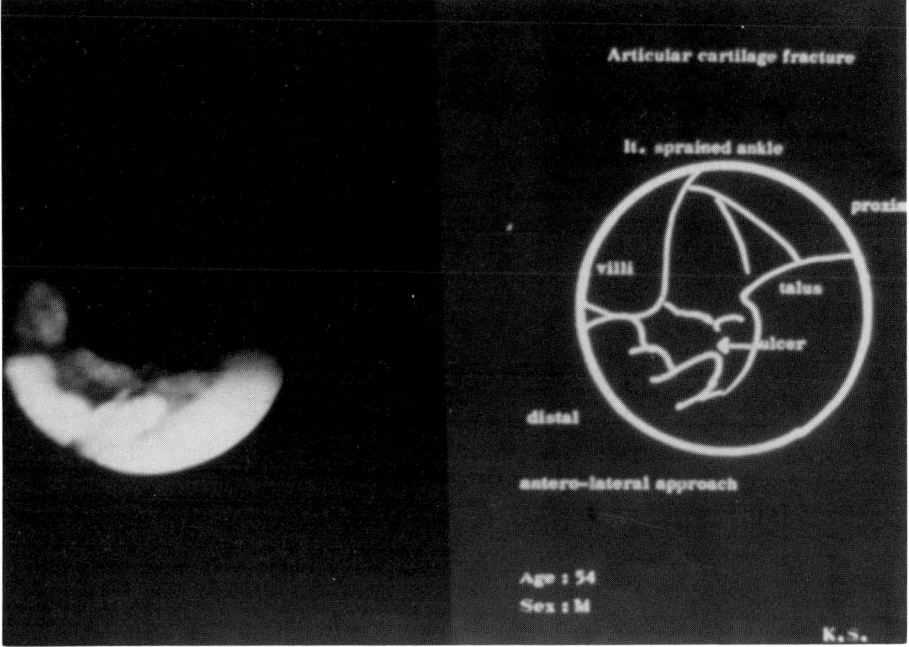

Figure 1-4. This illustration shows an intra-articular cartilage fracture.

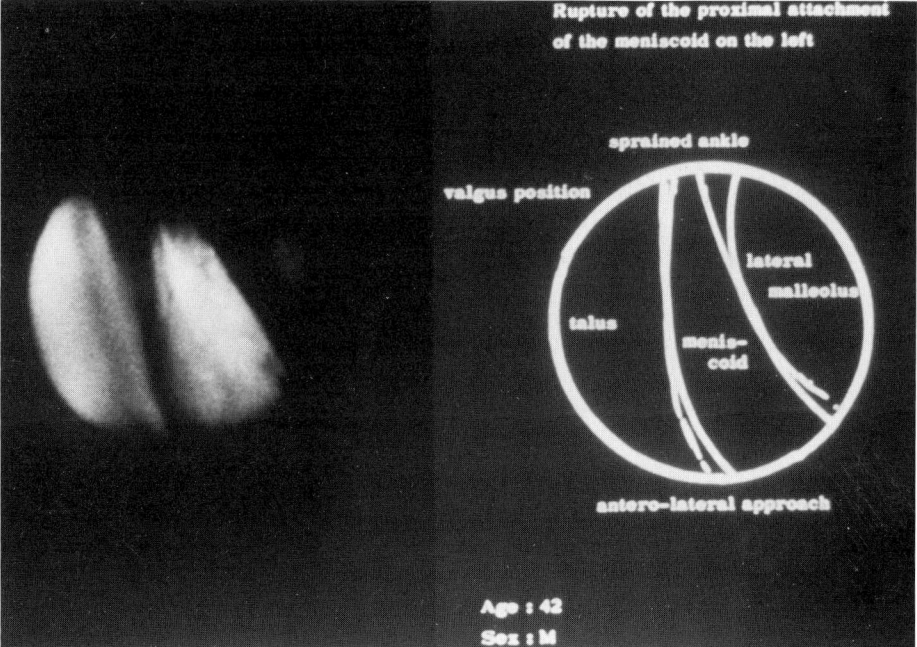
Figure 1-5. The meniscoid is again shown in this illustration of a sprained ankle.

portion of the joint, including lesions of the posterior dome of the talus and tibial plafond, was often difficult to visualize or treat satisfactorily.

Shortly thereafter, by the early 1980s, progress in ankle arthroscopy had reached the point that some lesions, such as chondral fragments, loose bodies, osteochondritis, chondral defects, and chronic synovitis, could be evaluated and probed in the anterior compartment and occasionally in the midcompartment. Arthroscopic biopsies were also obtained.

Later, when the large diameter arthroscopes became of more practical use, particularly in the ankle joint, one could see far better. Portals other than the anterolateral and anteromedial, which were originally used, were advocated, such as the posterolateral and the anterocentral portal. These were soon developed and employed by Drez, Guhl, and Gollehan.[4,5] This information was published in the *Sports Medicine Clinics of North America, The Journal of Foot and Ankle Surgery*, 1983, and by Gollehan[6] in *Contemporary Orthopedics*, 1984. The authors further described the technique of ankle arthroscopy and enlarged the indications, and further defined the complications and contraindications. This material was also presented at the 1981 Foot and Ankle Society's annual meeting in Las Vegas by Drez and Guhl[16] (and in a symposium by Schneider, Guhl, Ferkle, and Andrews in 1987).

Arthroscopic surgery of the ankle was demonstrated by Schonholtz, Guhl, and Andrews at various arthroscopic courses and seminars. Procedures were performed under significant restrictions because of the configuration of the ankle joint and tight ligaments. These limitations are mentioned in several textbooks on ankle surgery.[7,8]

In the early 1980s Johnson[3] described the use of the staple in fixing or

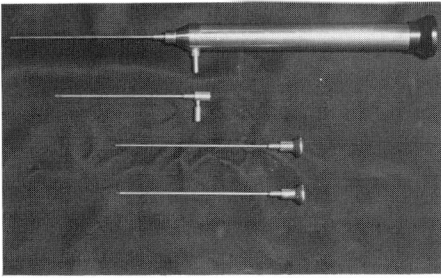

Figure 1-6. The needlescope was originally used in the ankle joint. Utilization of the larger arthroscopes in these joints was not appreciated at that time.

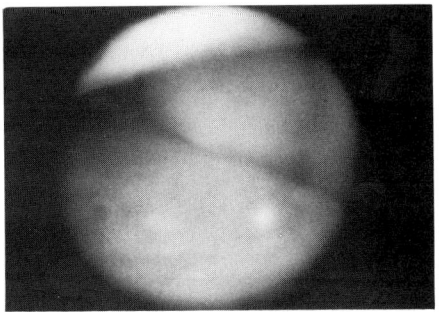

Figure 1-7. Inside view of the ankle taken through a 2.2 needlescope.

repairing the avulsed anterotalofibular ligaments arthroscopically to restore anterior and lateral stability. Hawkins[9] also described and reported his technique for this problem. Schneider,[10] Morgan,[11] and others described a small number of cases of ankle arthrodesis done arthroscopically. This seems to be a logical procedure. Parisien[12] of New York Hospital for Bone and Joint Surgery has done a significant amount of work on arthroscopy of the ankle as well as the talocalcaneal joint. His techniques have been described in *Contemporary Orthopedics*, 1982. He also reported his results for arthroscopic treatment of chondral defects at the meeting of the American Orthopedic Society for Sports Medicine in Nashville, Tennessee in June 1985. He and others have also developed several new instruments for performing arthroscopic surgery of the ankle.

There still was dissatisfaction with methods available to date for performing adequate diagnostic and operative arthroscopy of the ankle and particularly with methods for triangulating to perform surgery in that joint. Taking this into account, the distraction method was applied to the ankle joint. Based on Henning's[15] experience in the knee with this method, it seemed logical that this would be a safe procedure to apply to the ankle. Further work was done in the laboratory on amputation specimens. The procedure's safety was firmly established by careful documented followup and clinical trials of the cases in the second series. The transmalleolar approaches for drilling, debriding, and abrading defects in the midportion and posterior portion of the ankle joint were added to the distraction method. These areas at times could not be safely reached by the usual approaches. The original distractor, with modifications for the ankle joint, was developed in 1984. Several subsequent prototypes were manufactured, until the currently commercially available final product was made. It was later learned that Patel[13] had done similar work in ankle distraction in the anatomy laboratory.

In 1985 this author initiated the use of the ankle holder for better positioning of the patient and utilization of the portals. Further work was done with small reamers and jigs for utilizing other approaches.

Early experience was described by the author[14] in a preliminary report in *Orthopedics*, 1986. This method was shown in an exhibit at the American Academy of Orthopedic Surgeons in February 1986. The results were presented as an instructional course at the 1986 annual meeting of the Arthroscopy Association of North America, the 1986 American Orthopaedic Society of Sports Medicine annual meeting, and subsequent courses. In addition to the surgical procedures mentioned earlier, a more satisfying method of doing a complete evaluation of the ankle joint was obtained. Osteochondral and chondral lesions and defects could be better diagnosed and treated. A superior awareness of synovial lesions, such as the meniscoid of the ankle, adhesions, and the synovial impingement syndrome, developed. The development of new instruments, plus the distractor, ankle holder, transmalleolar approaches, and further utilization of the posterior approaches, now open the door for complete arthroscopic access to the ankle for diagnosis and treatment.

References

1. Ikeuchi H: Personal Communication.
2. Wolin I, Glassman F, Sideman S, et al: Internal Derangement of the Talofibular Joint of the Ankle. Surg Gyn & Ob 91:193-200, 1951.
3. Johnson L: Personal Communication.
4. Drez D, Guhl J, Gollehan DL: Ankle Arthroscopy: Technique and Indications. J Foot & Ankle 2:138-142, 1981.
5. Drez D, Guhl JF, Gollehan DL: Ankle Arthroscopy: Technique and Indications. Clin in Sports Med 1(1):35-45, 1982.
6. Gollehan DL, Drez D: Ankle Arthroscopy: Approach and Technique. Con Orth 6:1150-1152, 1983.
7. Leach DL, Yaplan IG, Segal D: Ankle Injuries. New York, Churchill Livingstone, 1983.
8. Kelikian H: Disorders of the Ankle. Philadelphia, W.B. Saunders Company, 1985.
9. Hawkins R: Arthroscopic Reconstruction for Chronic Lateral Instability of the Ankle. In: Arthroscopic Surgery Update. Rockville, Aspen, 1985, 175-181.
10. Schneider D:Personal Communication, 1985.
11. Morgan C: Personal Communication, 1986.
12. Parisien JS: Arthroscopy of the Ankle: State of the Art. Con Orth 5:21-27, 1982.
13. Patel D: Personal Communication.
14. Guhl J: Arthroscopic Advances: New Techniques for Arthroscopic Surgery of the Ankle: A preliminary report. Orth 9(2):261-269, 1986.
15. Hennings: Personal Communication, 1983.
16. Drez D, Guhl, JF: Annual Meeting, American Foot and Ankle Society, Las Vegas, 1981.

CHAPTER 2

GROSS ANATOMY OF THE ANKLE JOINT

Michael Harty, M.D., M.Ch., F.R.C.S. (Eng)

Motion and loading of the ankle joint occurs in all forms of human locomotion. Even today the ankle joint is the recipient of many traumatic insults and pathologic changes. To compensate for the absence of protective overlying muscles, the ankle joint has thick, strong ligaments firmly attached to the medial and lateral malleoli. Arthroscopy has opened a new concept of basic articular anatomy. The clear, close up, and enlarged image provides an excellent view of the joint walls and contents. In addition, subtle biological changes can be appreciated by instrument palpitation under direct observation. However, visualization of the joint cavity necessitates penetration of the overlying tissues such as skin, fascia, capsule, synovial membrane, and the avoidance of vital structures like nerves, blood vessels, and tendons.

Surface Anatomy

As in all joint approaches, the fixed palpable bony points provide the major landmarks and must be kept in mind in all stages of operative intervention.[4] The two malleoli covered by skin and fascia provide the salient bony features. The tip of the lateral malleolus is 2cm distal and 2cm posterior to the medial malleolus, and the anterior joint line is 2cm proximal to the latter. Anteriorly the joint is relatively superficial, being separated from the skin by the cutaneous nerves and veins in the subcutaneous fascia, the long extensor tendons, the dorsal neurovascular bundle, and the joint capsule (Figure 2-1).[3] The tendons are easily identified during active dorsiflexion. Inversion and plantar flexion displace them medially to allow palpation of the anterior lateral talar dome and joint line situated anteromedial to the lateral malleolus. The subcutaneous layer contains some sensitive and vulnerable

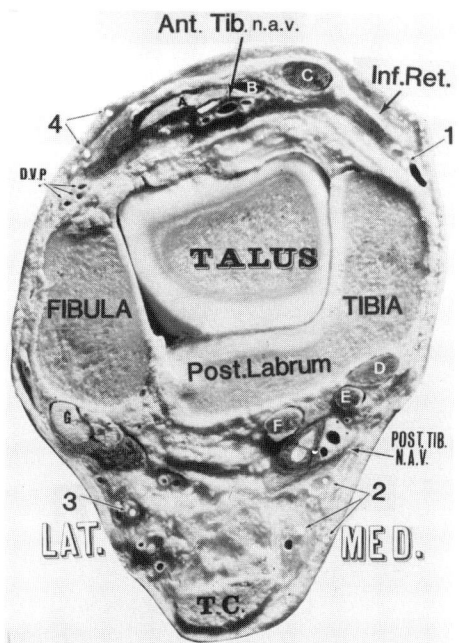

Figure 2-1. A transverse section through the talar dome. (a) Peroneus tertius and extensor digitorum longus; (b) Extensor hallucis longus; (c) Tibialis anterior; (d) Tibialis posterior; (e) Flexor digitorum longus; (f) Flexor hallucis longus; (g) Peronei; (1) Saphenous nerve and vein; (2) Medial calcaneal nerves; (3) Sural nerve and veins; (4) Cutaneous branches of superficial peroneal nerve, and dorsal venous plexus.
Adapted from Ankle Arthroscopy. Orth 8(12):1538, 1985[3].

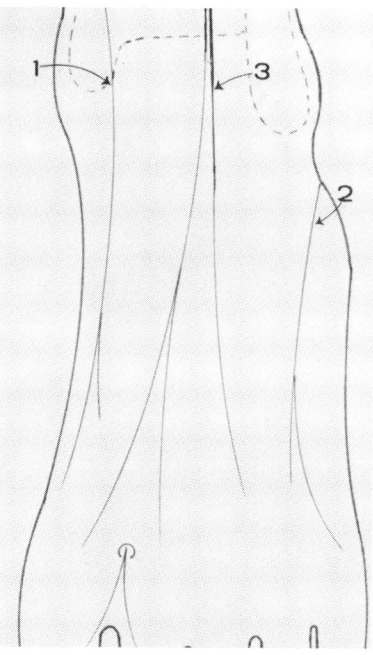

Figure 2-2. Dorsum of left foot showing cutaneous innervation. (1) Saphenous nerve; (2) Sural nerve; (3) Superficial peroneal nerve.

nerves, many with accompanying veins (Figure 2-2). The saphenous nerve with the great saphenous vein passes over the anterior edge of the medial malleolus (Figure 2-1). Note that all the extensor tendons to the dorsum of the foot pass on the medial side of the tibiofibular joint. Posteromedially, the tarsal tunnel carries the only neurovascular bundle to the sole of the foot, and the sensory nerves to the heel which are found in the subcutaneous layer (Figure 2-1).

Posterolaterally, the sural nerve with the short saphenous venous plexus lies behind the lateral malleolus. The terminal cutaneous branches to the superficial peroneal nerve with the dorsal venous plexus cross anteriorly to reach the dorsum of the foot (Figure 2-2). Posteriorly, the joint is more deeply situated, being covered posteromedially by the long flexor (plantar flexor tendons) and the neurovascular bundle to the sole. Posterolaterally, the tendons of the peroneus longus and brevis have moved behind the lateral malleolus. In addition, 3cm to 4cm of fibro fatty tissue intervene between these tendons and the tendo calcaneus (Figure 2-1). The posterior tendons are firmly tethered in their sheaths and do not displace readily. However, about 2cm of the posterolateral capsule between the tendons of the peronei and the flexor hallucis longus are covered by fibrous tissues and skin.

Bones

The close, overhanging canopy formed by the malleoli and tibial articular margins, combined with strong collateral ligaments, restrict distention of the ankle joint. The posterior articular margin of the tibia projects 3mm to 6mm more distally than the corresponding anterior margin. This posterior flange is further reinforced by the firmly attached transverse ligament (vide infra). The anterior articular margin lies approximately in the horizontal plane, except at its junction with the medial malleolus where it recedes proximally for 3mm to 5mm (Figure 2-3). This notch, illustrated without comment in older anatomy texts rarely shows on anteroposterior roentgenograms because it is hidden by the straight posterior articular flange, but it does provide the arthroscopist with the extra space needed to slip the instrument past the medial margin of the talar trochlear surface. In the distal 5cm (2 inches) of the leg, the anterior tibial artery and the deep peroneal nerve have moved from the interosseous membrane toward the anterior tibial margin. Transfixing pins in the distal 10cm (4 inches) of the leg may impinge on this neurovascular bundle (Figure 2-4).

At the inferior tibiofibular fibrous joint, the fibula is held firmly in the tibial groove by the strong interosseous ligament. A small synovial-lined recess reaches proximally for a distance of about 5mm and it may contain a synovial fold.

Talus

The talar dome or trochlear surface, wider anteriorly than posteriorly, is

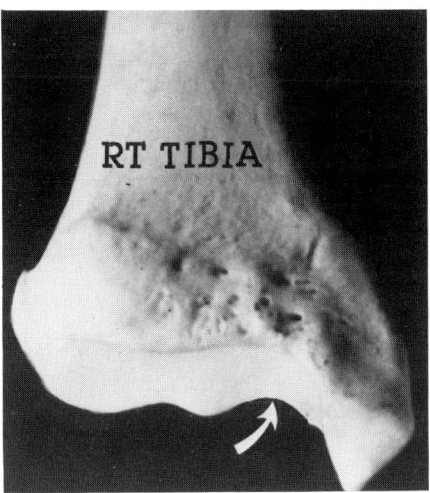

Figure 2-3. The anterior articular margin of the tibia. Note the bony retraction at medial side (arrow).

convex in the sagittal plane and slightly concave in the coronal plane. This transverse concavity throws the collateral articular margins into prominence and is an etiologic factor in producing transcondylar fractures of the talar dome. Of these, 57% are found on the medial and commonly posterior edge, while 43% occur on the central area of the lateral edge.[1] The medial ligaments of the ankle and knee are strong, dense, and inelastic, making the posteromedial corner of both joints difficult to visualize from an anterior approach, as in all anatomical structures minor variations are encountered. The flatter convex dome, especially in a looser joint, allows more room for manipulation of the arthroscope, as does the deeper transverse depression, which is utilized during the central anterior approaches. The central area of the calcaneous is 3cm distal and posterior to the tip of the lateral malleolus (Figure 2-5). A distraction pin in this area avoids the neurovascular bundle to the sole and the peroneal tendons, but a pin placed near the posterior tubercle may force the foot into dorsiflexion.

Ligaments

The medial malleolus overhangs the talar dome and provides firm anchorage for the thick, strong, deltoid ligament, which fans distally to the talus, the calcaneous, the spring ligament, and the navicular. The lateral malleolus, projecting even more distally, gives attachment to the calcano fibular ligament, the posterior talofibular ligament, and the posterior

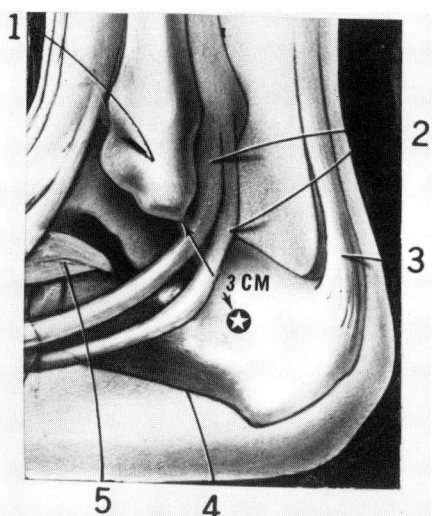

Figure 2-5. The lateral aspect of the left heel and ankle, showing the recommended site for insertion of a distraction pin. (1) Lateral malleolus; (2) Peronei tendons; (3) Tendo calcaneus; (4) Os calcis; (5) Extensor digitorum brevis. Adapted from Foot Disorders: Medical and Surgical Management. Giannestras J. Lea & Fibiger, 1973, 24-58.[5]

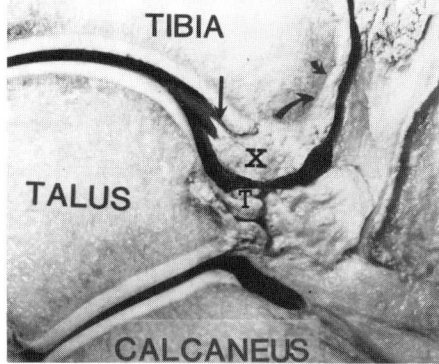

Figure 2-6. "X" indicates the transverse ligament as a distal and deeper condensation of the posterior inferior tibiofibular ligament (curved arrows). Two small synovial folds or plicas (straight arrows). "T" shows the posterior talofibular ligament.

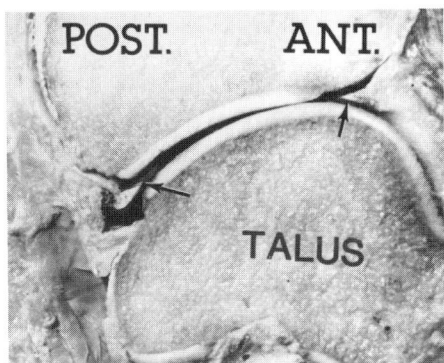
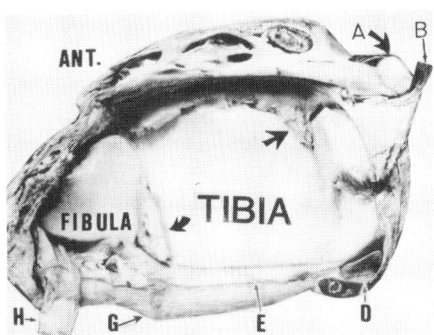

Figure 2-7. The anterior and posterior synovial plicas.

Figure 2-8. An interior view of the right tibiofibular mortice. (a) Tibialis anterior; (b) Deltoid ligament; (d) Tibialis posterior; (e) Transverse tibiofibular ligament; (g) Posteroinferior tibiofibular ligament; (h) Calcano fibular ligament. Fatty synovial fold in syndesmosis (curved arrows). Fat pad in anterior tibial notch (straight arrow) c.f. Figure 2-3.

inferior tibiofibular ligament with its most deeply placed inferior condensation, designated the transverse ligament (Figure 2-6). This synovial-covered ligament is more obvious from the anterior (joint) aspect. It increases the posterior tibial flange, deepens the plafond, and helps prevent posterior talar displacement during sudden landing on the forefoot. In about 70% of the older specimens seen in anatomy laboratories, the synovial covering is frayed or even absent. During plantar flexion, the transverse ligament appears as a horizontal ridge squeezed between the posterior articular tibial margin and the posterior talofibular ligament. However, during dorsiflexion, with or without joint distraction, the posterior talofibular ligament moves distally to expose a synovial-lined cul-de-sac. The floor of this recess may occasionally show a thin capsular condensation — the tibial slip stretching from the lateral end of the posterior talofibular ligament to the medial end of the transverse ligament (See Figures 3-18 and 9-17). It should be noted that this slip, when present, is extrasynovial. It is more obvious from the anterior arthroscopic approaches, but is not seen as readily from the posterolateral portal.

Synovial folds or plicas are an indispensible part of the chondrosynovial junction in all movable joints.[2] They must be loose, pliable, and elastic in order to allow synovial slide on the capsule or bone. They fill the dead space and often contain fat lobules (plicae adiposae or Haversian fat pads).

They are found between the synovial membrane and the overlying capsule or intra-articular bones. The enlarged image provided by the arthroscope has given a new emphasis to these synovial plicas. In the ankle joint, they are seen at the anterior and posterior tibiotalar junctions (Figure 2-7), and projecting from the lower end of the inferior tibiofibular syndesmosis (Figure 2-8). The posterior plica is simply the synovial-covered transverse ligament,

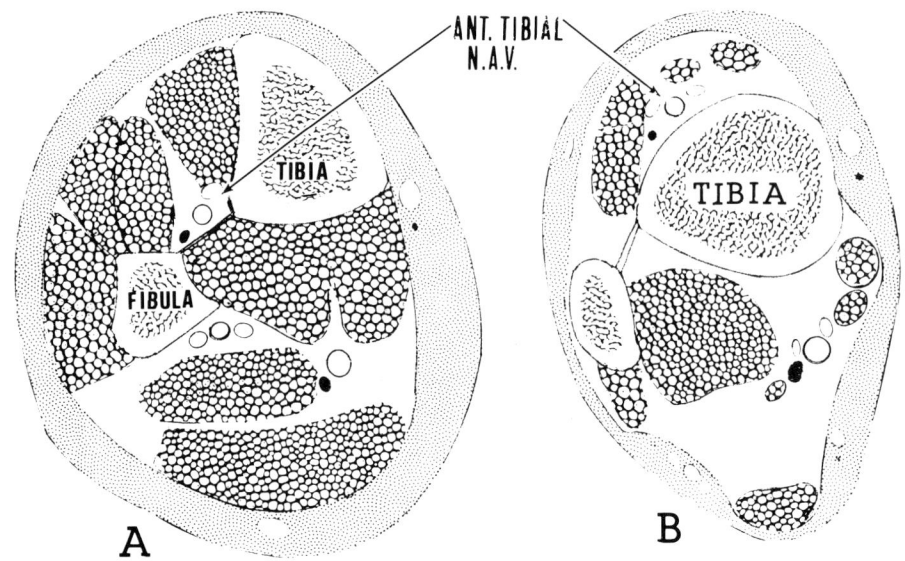

Figure 2-4. A transverse section of the distal leg. (a) 10cm (4 inches) proximal to the ankle joint. The neural vascular bundle is safely protected between the tibia and fibula; (b) 5cm (2 inches) proximal to the ankle joint.

but, occasionally, in dorsiflexion, it may appear as a double fold, just to complicate the arthroscopic view (Figure 2-6).

Arthrograms have demonstrated distensible articular recesses on the dorsum of the talar neck anterior to the talar dome, and, in 25% of cases, the contrast medicine reaches the posterior talocalcaneal joint.

Sharp distention is limited to skin incisions in order to avoid damage to cutaneous nerves, blood vessels, and tendons. The location and size of the pathologic lesions, as well as the position of the more important anatomic structures, will often dictate the type and site of the arthroscopic or surgical approach. As in all joint examinations, carefully thought out movements and instrument manipulation help to expose hidden recesses of the synovial cavity.

References

1. Berndt AL, Harty M: Transcondylar Fractures (osteochondritis dissecans). J of Bone & Joint Surg 41:988-1020, 1959.
2. Harty M, Joyce JJ III: Synovial Folds in the Knee Joint. Orth Rev 6:10, 1977.
3. Harty M: Ankle Arthroscopy, Anatomical Features. Orth 8(12):1538-1540, 1985.
4. Joyce JJ III, Harty M: Orthopaedic Approaches. Baltimore, Williams & Wilkins, 1961.
5. Giannestras J: Heart Fribiger Foot Disorders: Medical & Surgical Management, 1973, 24-58.

CHAPTER 3

ARTHROSCOPIC ANATOMY

Dinesh Patel, M.D.
James F. Guhl, M.D.

A knowledge of anatomy, both gross and arthroscopic, is essential to understand the pathological entities of any joint. It is also necessary to employ properly the arthroscopic approaches or portals when utilizing triangulation and effectively performing surgery.

The internal anatomy of the ankle is presented in this chapter with emphasis placed on the structures one should recognize arthroscopically to interpret pathology properly. This is done by illustrating the views to which one must become accustomed when employing the recommended portals. The arthroscopic anatomy seen in the normal (stable) ankle joint, as compared to that seen with the use of mechanical distraction, is emphasized. The 5mm, 25 degree or 30 degree oblique arthroscope is used routinely. The 5mm, 70 degree arthroscope and the 2.5mm are used for special indications.

In the earlier publications by Drez, Guhl, and Gollahan,[1,3] the ankle joint has been subdivided into the anterior, anterolateral, and anteromedial compartments, and also into the posterior, posterolateral and posteromedial chambers (Figures 3-1 and 3-2). The points of anatomy to be noted in these areas are shown in the accompanying illustrations (Figures 3-3 and 3-4). Arthroscopic views are presented as seen on the video monitor (Figures 3-5 through 3-12). Comparative views with mechanical distraction also are shown (Figures 3-13 and 3-14).

Structures encompassing or comprising the ankle joint itself are the distal articular surface of the tibia or plafond (roof or vault), the articular surface of the talus, with its medial and lateral articular malleolar surfaces, and the articular surface of the medial malleolus and fibula. The joint is divided into the distal tibiofibular joint with its synovial recess (Figure 3-15), the middle or

ANTERIOR JOINT CAVITY
1. Anterior compartment
2. Anterolateral compartment
3. Anteromedial compartment

Figure 3-1. Drez D, Guhl JF, Gollehan DL: J of Foot & Ankle Surg, 1981.

POSTERIOR JOINT CAVITY
1. Posterior compartment
2. Posterolateral compartment
3. Posteromedial compartment

Figure 3-2. Drez, et al.

ANTERIOR JOINT CAVITY
I Anterior Compartment
Anterior-superior aspect proper T-T joint
II Anterolateral Compartment
Anterior T-F ligament
Anterior aspect distal T-F joint
Anterior aspect lateral T-M space
III Anteromedial Compartment
Anterior aspect medial T-M space

Figure 3-3. Drez, et al.

POSTERIOR JOINT CAVITY
I Posterior Compartment
Post-superior aspect proper T-T joint
II Posterolateral Compartment
Post. T-F ligament
Post. aspect distal T-F joint
Post. aspect lateral T-M space
III Posteromedial Compartment
Post. aspect medial T-M space

Figure 3-4. Drez, et al.

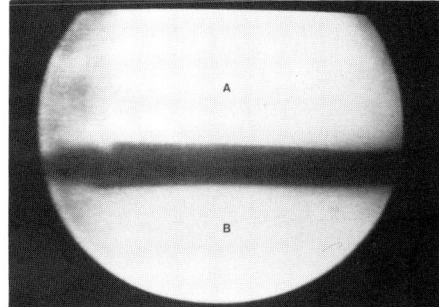

Figure 3-5. The anterior talofibular ligament (A) as seen in the video arthroscopic views of the anterior inferior aspect of the distal talofibular joint. B, fibula; C, talus. Drez, et al.

Figure 3-6. Video arthroscopic view of the anterior joint cavity, showing the tibia (A, anterior lip—or edge—of tibia) above and anterior portion of the talar dome (B) below, as seen without mechanical distraction. Drez, et al.

proper tibial talar joint (talocrural joint), the medial and lateral talomalleolar joints, plus the anterior and posterior joint pouches or recesses (Figure 3-16).

Emphasis is placed on structures such as the anterior talofibular ligament, the ridge or anterior edge or lip of the talus, the synovial recess of the distal tibiofibular joint, peroneal tendons and their tenosynovial sheaths, the transverse tibiofibular ligament (and/or tibial slip), and the posterior talofibular ligament (Figures 3-17 through 3-19). The latter three structures are difficult and at times impossible to observe in many ankles from the anterior

Arthroscopic Anatomy   15

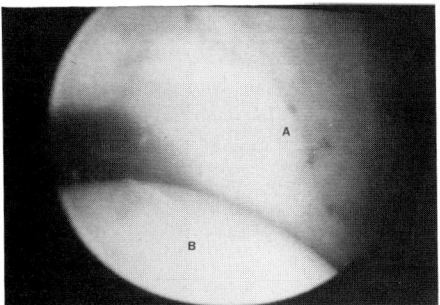

Figure 3-7. Video arthroscopic view of the medial malleolus (A) at the anterior aspect of the talomalleolar space. B, dome of talus. Drez, et al.

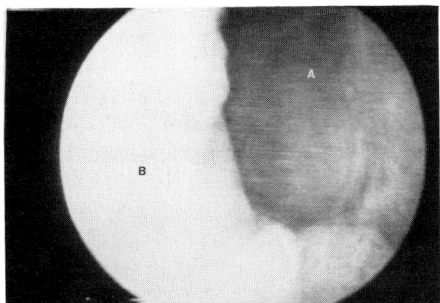

Figure 3-8. Video arthroscopic view of the neck of the talus in the anterior joint cavity. Note the anterior capsule (A) shown through the synovial membrane on the right. B, anterior neck of talus. Drez, et al.

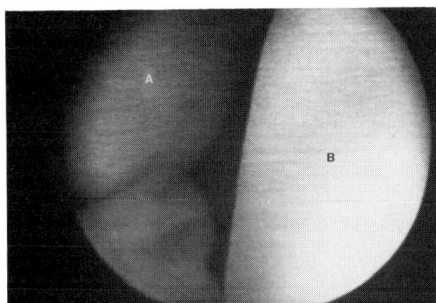

Figure 3-9. A video arthroscopic view of the posterior joint cavity from the posterolateral portal. The medial malleolus (A) is shown on the left and the posterior medial portion of the dome of the talus (B) on the right. Drez, et al.

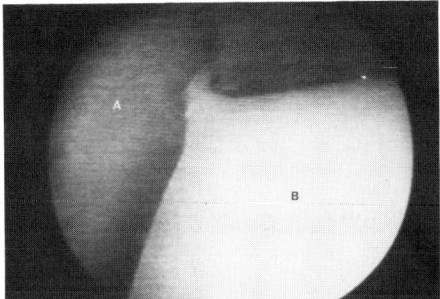

Figure 3-10. The same view as the arthroscope is moved to a superior position. The medial malleolus (A) is on the left and the plafond is above. B, posteromedial dome of talus. Drez, et al.

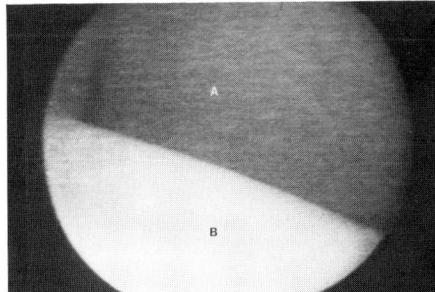

Figure 3-11. In this video arthroscopic view, the posterior 60% to 70% of the plafond (A) can be seen without distraction, while the posterior 50% of the articular surface of the dome of the talus (B) can be examined. Drez, et al.

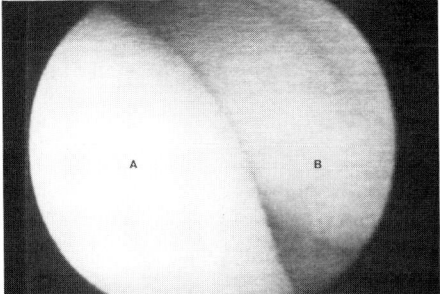

Figure 3-12. The arthroscope has been moved laterally and downward, showing the posterior lateral articular surface of the talus (A) and a posterior view of the distal fibula (B) on the right. Drez, et al.

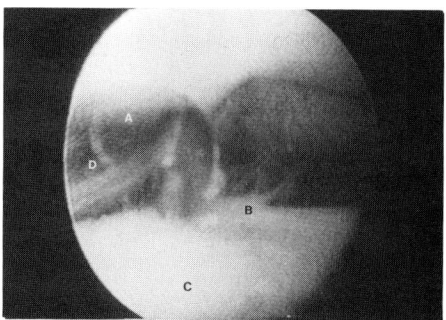

Figure 3-13. An arthroscopic view of the left ankle with distraction as seen on the video monitor through the anterolateral portal. Note the medial malleolus (A) on the left and the chondral defect (B) of the talus. C, dome of talus; D, probe.

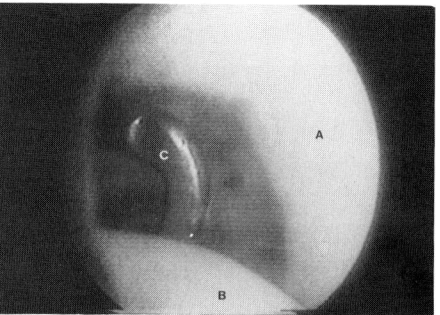

Figure 3-14. An arthroscopic view of the same ankle with distraction as viewed from the posterolateral portal. Note the medial malleolus (A) now on the right, the posterior medial talar dome (B), and the probe (C).

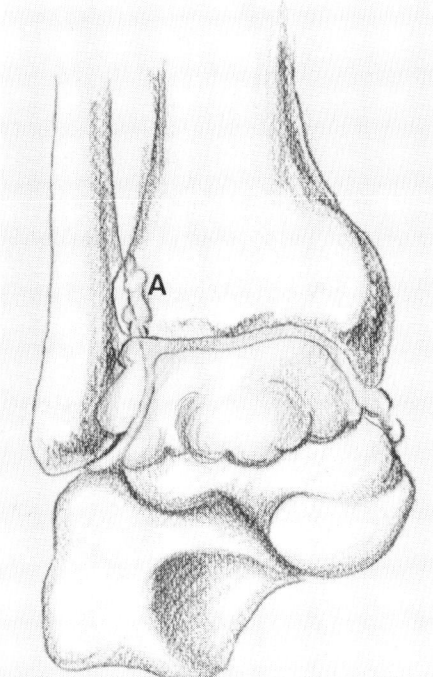

Figure 3-15. The anterior ankle, showing the superior synovial recess (A) of the distal tibiofibular joint communicating with the lateral talofibular joint. (Modified from Kelikian.)

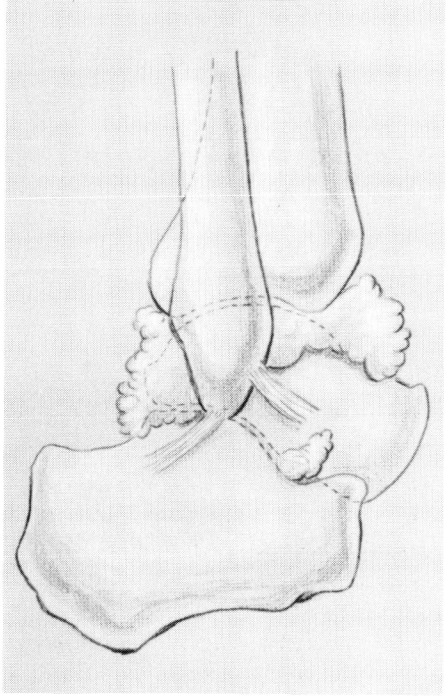

Figure 3-16. This illustration of the lateral aspect of the ankle joint depicts the anterior and posterior synovial recesses. The extent of these synovial cavities should be kept in mind when interpreting arthrograms. Also note the proximity of the talotibial joint and the subtalar joint in the posterior recess. Care should be taken not to insert the arthroscope into the wrong joint when employing the posterior approaches.

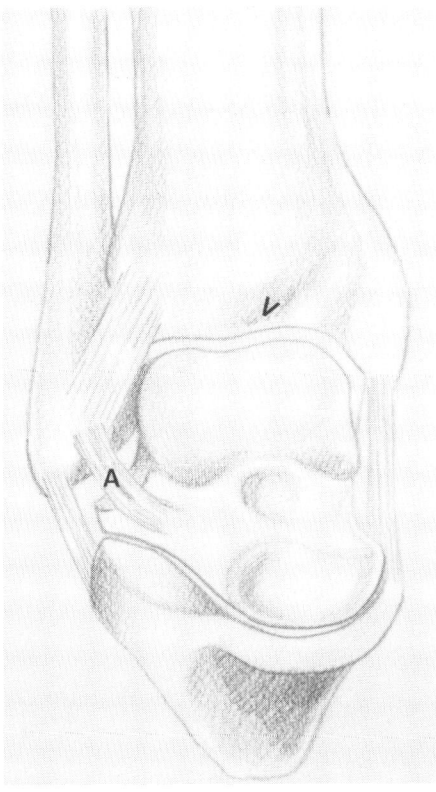

Figure 3-17. Shown is the relationship of the anterior talofibular ligament (A) to the ankle joint (arrow). (Modified from Kelikian.)

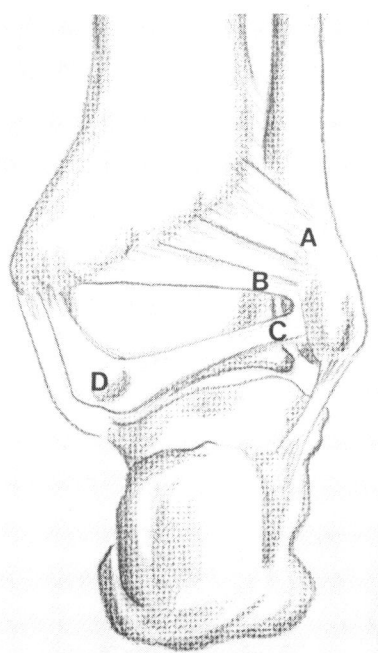

Figure 3-18. This view of the posterior ankle joint illustrates the relationship of ligaments in that area. Note the posterior tibiofibular ligament (A), transverse tibiofibular ligament (B), the posterior talofibular ligament (C), the os trigonum (D). (Modified from Kelikian.) Figure 9-16 shows the same diagram with the addition of the tibial slip.

approaches without adequate (mechanical) distraction. These entities are seen through the synovial membrane or lining of the joint. Prior to the utilization of arthroscopy, they were not seen from this vantage point. They cannot be observed from the posterolateral portal (with the exception, to some degree, of the transverse tibiofibular ligament), since they are extraarticular in location. (Figures 3-20 through 3-22). Pathology is believed to have occurred (or can develop from or in conjunction with) all of these structures, as described in Chapter IX.

The lateral synovial or soft tissue impingement originates from the synovial recess of the distal tibiofibular joint and adheres to the undersurface of the interosseous membrane. This appears to be caused by trauma, usually a moderate sprain or minimal fracture, and is often associated with a disruption of the anterior capsule and ligamentous tissue, as well as of the synovial tissue. Interarticular ganglia may develop from the tenosynovial sheaths of the peroneal tendons. The anterior tibial lip is the point of origin of the anterior osteophyte or anterior impingement, which is often intraarticular and at times incorporated in the anterior capsule. An understanding and appreciation of these normal structures will then give the arthroscopic surgeon a point of reference when excising pathological lesions.

Figure 3-19. The lateral ankle joint, showing ligaments. (A) posterior talofibular ligament, (B) anterior talofibular ligament, (C) calcaneal.

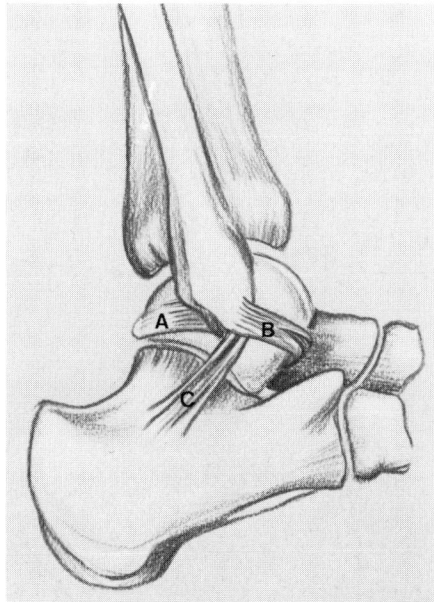

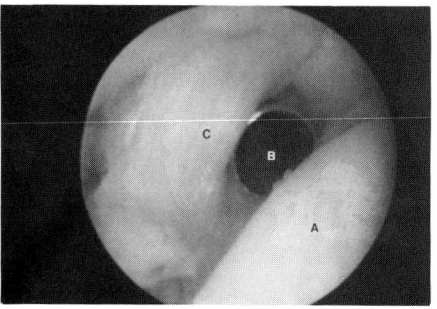

Figure 3-20. A video arthroscopic view from the anterolateral portal. The posterolateral aspect of the dome of the talus (A) is to the lower right. The cannula (B) for the arthroscope can be seen below the transverse tibiofibular ligament (C), between it and the talus.

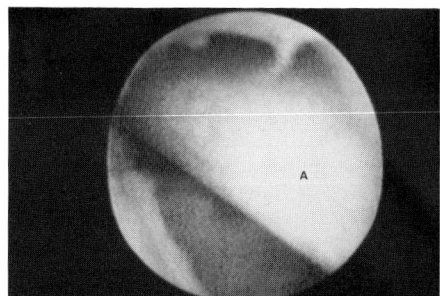

Figure 3-21. A view of the posterior edge of the transverse tibiofibular ligament (A) as seen from an arthroscope placed in the cannula through the posterolateral portal.

The anterior talofibular ligament is the first structure on the lateral side of the ankle to be ruptured in an ankle sprain. It can be easily seen in the normal joint, but it is somewhat more difficult to recognize when it is the cause of pathology and one is considering arthroscopic stabilization of the ankle[4] (Figures 3-23 and 3-24). Also, when debriding a chronic synovitis from the anterior compartment or recess, one should take care to identify it and not cause injury. The same is true of the anterior division of the deltoid ligament on the medial side. The transverse tibiofibular ligament should be noted and appreciated (Figure 3-25). It can vary in size or be a double structure.(Figure 3-26) Differentiation must be made between it and an adhesion, or the meniscus, or synovial folds of the posterior joint recess. It is

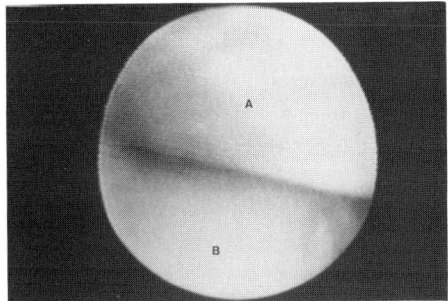

Figure 3-22. The same video arthroscopic view as above, with the arthroscope passed under the transverse tibiofibular ligament (A) from the posterolateral approach. The talus (B) is below.

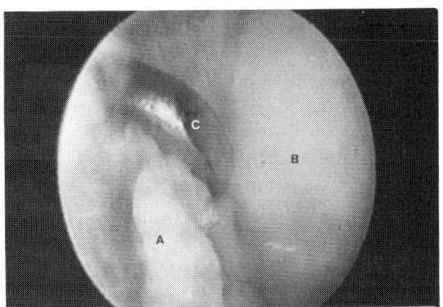

Figure 3-23. A video arthroscopic view of the anterior talofibular ligament (A) in its pathological form after being avulsed from the talus (B). C, probe.

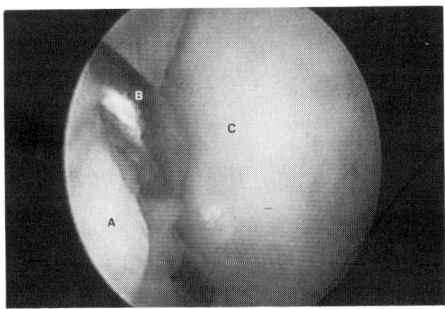

Figure 3-24. The same video arthroscopic view as the arthroscope scans further down, showing the site of its previous attachment. A, avulsed anterior talofibular ligament; B, talus; C, probe.

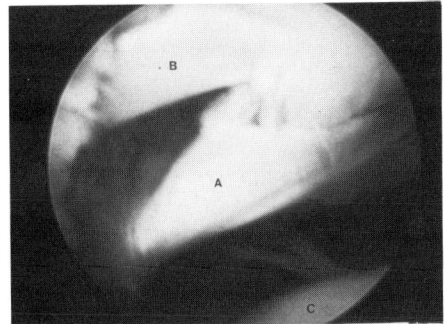

Figure 3-25. A 35mm arthroscopic view of the transverse tibiofibular ligament (A) as seen from the anterolateral portal. B, tibia; C, talus.

also believed by some authorities that it may hypertrophy secondary to trauma, thus becoming pathological and a source or cause of chronic pain. It therefore could require partial excision arthroscopically (Chapter IX). This structure originates from the distal fibula adjacent and, proximal to the origin of the posterior talofibular ligament, and runs in an oblique fashion to the posterior tibia at its junction with the medial malleolus.

A similar structure, described by Ikeuchi[6] and Chen,[5] and referred to as a tibial slip in Chapter IX, is located just above the posterior talofibular ligament. It originates from the posterior talofibular ligament itself and extends obliquely to the posterior tibia. This variation is still not completely understood. Appreciation of the location of these anatomical entities is shown in Figures 3-18 and 9-16. The relationship of the transverse tibiofibular ligament and the posterior talofibular ligament is shown, as well as the separation that occurs in dorsiflexion of the ankle, as noted by Kelikian[7] (Figure 3-27). This, of course, is not seen arthroscopically. The posterior talofibular ligament was noted arthroscopically by Chen,[5] and he pointed out that it could become fibrosed or enlarged as a result of trauma and therefore be the cause

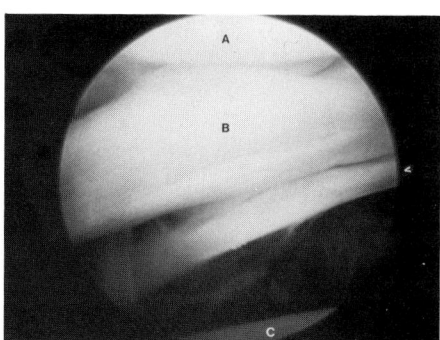

Figure 3-26. A similar arthroscopic view (35mm) of a double transverse tibiofibular ligament. The smaller structure is also referred to as the tibial slip (arrow). A, tibia; B, transverse tibiofibular ligament; C, talus.

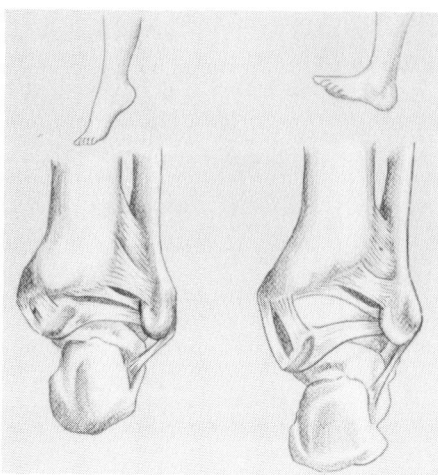

Figure 3-27. A posterior view of the ankle. This shows the relationship of the transverse tibiofibular ligament to the posterior talofibular ligament in full plantar flexion of the ankle as compared to dorsiflexion or extension. (Modified from Kelikian.)

of chronic ankle pain. This also may be amenable to partial arthroscopic excision for relief of chronic pain.

Another pathological structure in the ankle is the meniscoid (advanced form of the synovial impingement) in the lateral talofibular joint, as described by Wolin.[8] Anatomical variants can also become pathological, such as the true meniscus of the posterior ankle joint compartment, as well as the labrum, which occurs in some ankles. The latter two have been described by Hamilton[9] in Chapter VIII. An understanding of normal anatomy, as seen through the arthroscope, must be mastered so that one can recognize these aberrations.

The opening of the lateral talofibular joint anteriorly is covered by a cartilagenous plica, which was described by Chen (Figure 3-28). This has no functional or pathological significance as seen by this authors to date, but at times can be noted when arthroscoping the ankle.

Also, it should be further noted that the roof of the joint proper, or tibial plafond, is slightly convex in the coronal plane. There is a medial notch of the lower anterior lip, noted by Chen,[5] near its junction with the medial malleolus (Figure 3-29). He pointed out that the arthroscope may therefore be more easily passed into the joint proper from the anteromedial portal. The tip of the arthroscope can at times be inserted further in a loose joint or, with the use of a small telescope, reach the posterior recess easier than may be accomplished from the anterolateral approach.

While the talocrural joint proper has a convex plafond, it also has a concavity of the talar articular surface in the coronal plane. This is exaggerated in certain marsupials, such as the kangaroo, but is less so in man, although there it also varies to some degree (Figure 3-30). The authors have noted that because of this variation the larger 5mm arthroscope (or operating instruments) can be passed through the midjoint and further posterior when inserted through the anterocentral approach and with more ease when distraction is employed (Chapter VI). This is done with more difficulty from the anteromedial and anterolateral approaches because of the raised edges or "humps" of the medial or lateral talus. Triangulation consequently can be performed for carrying out surgery in the more posterior aspect of the joint from anterior. This is done best with the arthroscope anteromedial or anterolateral and the instruments inserted through the anterocentral portal. It was found that most ankles, even with pathology such as synovial impingement lesions or osteochondral defects, are relatively stable or tight and loose joints are in the minority. The mechanical distraction method thus allows greater access to the mid and posterior portion of the ankle joint when utilizing this combination of anterior portals, because of this anatomical configuration.

When the ankle joint is distracted sufficiently, about 70% to 80% of the talar dome can be seen from any of the anterior portals. In most cases the entire plafond can also be viewed. This allows ample room for both the diagnostic ability of the arthroscopist and for greater ease of performing surgery. If it is necessary to see the remainder of the dome, the 70 degree arthroscope can be inserted from the anterior portals or the posterolateral approach can be employed. Without this method only about the anterior 40% to 60% of the dome can be inspected from the anterior approaches, even with the foot and ankle in full plantar flexion. Also little more than the anterior edge of the tibia and a small part of the plafond can be viewed, except in loose joints.

The posterolateral portal is easier to utilize when distracting the ankle mechanically and employing the ankle holder. Triangulation can be accomplished from anterior-posterior or vice versa with this method (Chapter VI).

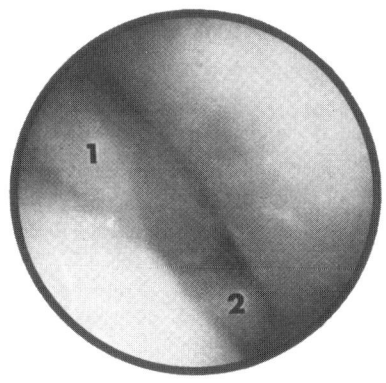

Figure 3-28. The cartilagenous plica, 1; at the superior entrance of the lateral talofibular joint is shown, as well as the posterior talofibular ligament, 2; located more posteriorly. From Chen (Arthroscopy of Small Joints, Watanabe) with permission.

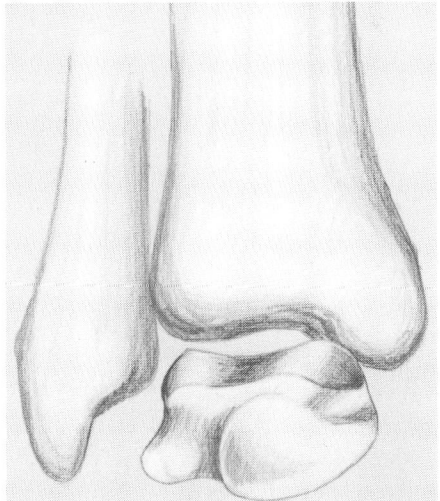

Figure 3-29. This illustration of the anterior ankle shows the notch at the junction of the anterior tibial lip and the medial malleolus.

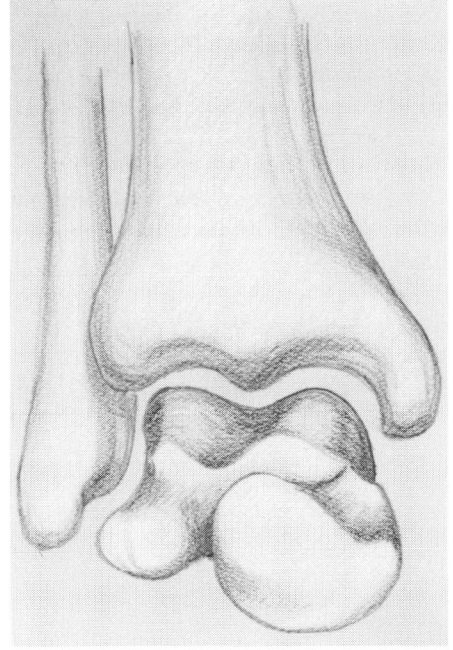

Figure 3-30. An early mammalian form of the talocrural joint (tibiotalar joint proper). The convex plafond and the concavity of the talus are illustrated. This is of course less exaggerated in the human ankle. It tends to block the passage of the arthroscope in passing from the anterolateral and anteromedial portals to the more posterior aspect of the joint. However, with the joint distracted, the arthroscope or instruments can be passed posteriorly with greater ease, especially through the antero-central approach.

When examining the normal ankle joint with distraction as described, the entire surface of the articular cartilage can be evaluated and probed. This surface appears shiny, yellowish-white, glistening, and firm. Any variation, such as a dull appearance, discoloration, elevation or depression of the surface, softness or fibrillation, should be considered abnormal and recognized.

Conclusion

The above discussion has emphasized understanding and recognizing normal anatomical structures arthroscopically enhanced by mechanical distraction in order to distinguish them from abnormal variations and pathology to achieve better diagnostic acumen and more efficient and safer surgery.

References
1. Drez D, Guhl JF, Gollehan DL: Ankle Arthroscopy: Technique and Indications. J Foot & Ankle Surg 2: 138-142, 1981.
2. Drez D, Guhl JF, Gollehan DL: Ankle Arthroscopy: Technique and Indications. Clin in Sports Med 1(1): 35-45, 1982.
3. Gollehan DL, Drez D: Arthroscopic Surgery Update. McGinty J ed. 14(15): 161-173, Text; Aspen Systems Corporation, 1985.
4. Hawkins, RB: Arthroscopic Reconstruction for Chronic Lateral Instability of the Ankle in Arthroscopic Surgery Update. McGinty J. ed. Rockville, Aspen 1985, 175-181.

5. Chen Y: Arthroscopy of the Ankle Joint. In: Arthroscopy of Small Joints. New York. IGAKU-SHOIN, 1985, 104-128.
6. Ikeuchi H: Personal Communication, 1977.
7. Kelikian H: Disorders of the Ankle. Philadelphia, W.B. Saunders Company, 1985.
8. Wolin I, Glassman F, Sideman S: Internal Derangement of Talofibular Components of the Ankle. Surg Gyn and Ob 91: 193-200, 1950.
9. Hamilton W: Personal Communication, 1986.

CHAPTER 4

RADIOLOGICAL TECHNIQUES

C.F. Carrera, M.D.
James F. Guhl, M.D.

Conventional radiographic examination of the ankle, including at a minimum AP, lateral, and 20 degree internal oblique (mortise) projections, must be performed prior to ankle arthroscopy. The internal oblique view is particularly important because the dome of the talus is projected free of the overlying density from the malleoli. Stress films can be useful adjuncts to conventional x-rays, particularly when ligamentous damage may be part of the clinical complex. Some investigators consider stress films an essential part of the prearthroscopy routine.

Other radiological modalities may be useful in detecting occult pathology, evaluating the metabolic activity of a lesion, or providing more refined anatomic information. Radioisotope scanning is useful and sensitive for detecting occult lesions and also for establishing the presence of reparative activity at the site of the anatomic abnormality. Tomographic techniques, including conventional tomography, and particularly, computed tomography, provide exquisite anatomic discrimination of subtle lesions in the ankle joint, which may be obscured by an overlying density in conventional radiographic examinations. Magnetic resonance imaging (MR) is an exciting new technique that has received some attention in evaluating the ankle. The primary value of MR appears to be its ability to discriminate soft tissue densities such as the synovium and ligaments. While still experimental, MR may find a significant place in the work-up of ankle abnormalities.

The practical application of these techniques will be further discussed in the remainder of this chapter.

Conventional Radiography

Plain x-rays are useful for evaluating bony lesions in and about the ankle, as well as evaluating the development and position of the bones forming the ankle joint. Such lesions as fractures, osteochondral defects, degenerative changes, including joint narrowing and osteophytes, erosions, tumors, osteomyelitis, and osteochondritis dissecans are often well evaluated on conventional radiographic examination.

Osteochondral defects in the lateral talar dome are more easily seen with conventional radiographic projections than those involving the medial talus. Most lesions of the lateral dome are located in the middle or anterior third of the talus, which is the area best demonstrated on routine projections. In addition, displaced lesions are more common in the lateral dome than in the medial, making radiographic detection easier.

Lesions of the medial talar dome are more frequently undisplaced, and can be more difficult to detect. Subtle compression fractures are often difficult to visualize until resorption of a significant area of a subchondral plate has occurred. In addition, medial defects occur frequently in the posterior third of the talar dome and can be obscured on conventional radiographic examinations. Internal oblique projection with plantar flexion of the ankle and foot may be necessary to visualize these lesions.

Osteochondral fractures can sometimes be staged according to x-ray appearance. Stage I lesions are generally radiographically occult, since there

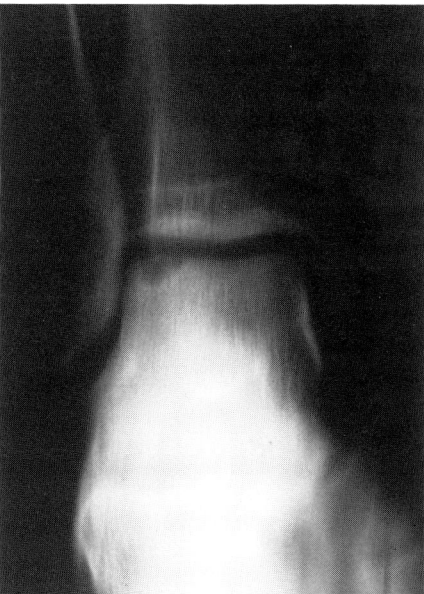

Figure 4-1. Mortise view (internal oblique) showing an osteochondritic lesion of the lateral talar dome that appears intact. At arthroscopy the articular cartilage was loose and partially separated (See Chapter X).

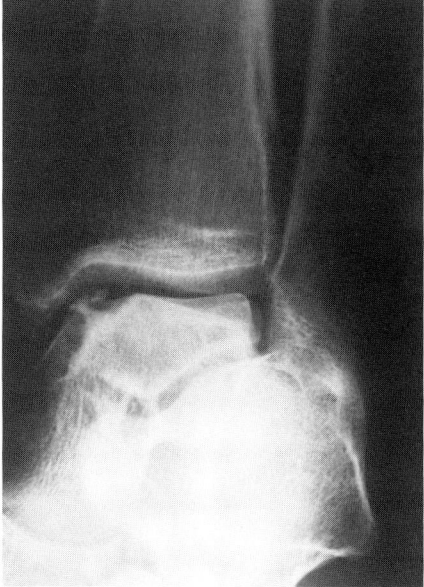

Figure 4-2. Mortise view showing an apparently separated osteochondritic lesion of the medial talus. The articular cartilage was completely intact and unaffected at arthroscopy.

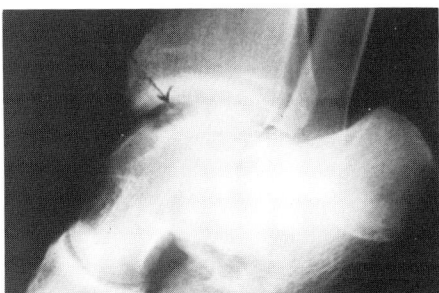

Figure 4-3. An off lateral view shows an osteochondritic lesion that was hard to appreciate on routine projections.

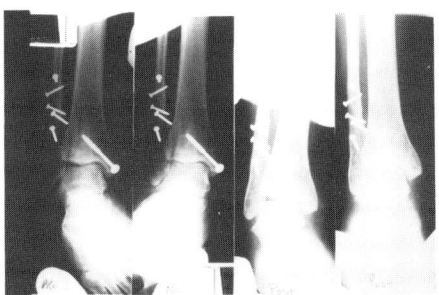

Figure 4-4. These AP stress films show no change in the talotibial angle pre-and postoperatively when distraction was employed. This finding occurred in each of the 38 cases followed by the author (JFG) when repeat stress x-rays were done. Stress views in the anterior-posterior plane also remained unchanged pre and postoperatively in several cases later in the series.

is no fracture of subchondral bone. Stage II lesions (incomplete subchondral fractures) and Stage III lesions (complete fractures with mild separation) can frequently be diagnosed on x-ray. Stage IV lesions are those with rotational displacement of the osteochondral fragment, a diagnosis which is occasionally apparent on x-ray when the separated fragment is completely incongruous within its bed.

It must be emphasized, however, that radiographic examination for staging of osteochondral defects is imperfect and should not be considered final without direct examination of the fracture site. Some lesions that appear to be relatively less displaced on x-ray examination can be arthroscopically documented as severely displaced; conversely, some lesions that appear seriously displaced on x-ray may prove to be much less abnormal at arthroscopy (Figures 4-1 and 4-2).

On occasion, additional obliquities of the ankle, as well as a range of dorsiflexion and plantar flexion positions of the foot, may be most useful in evaluating different areas of the talar dome (Figure 4-3). Unexplained clinical findings, bone scan abnormalities, and incompletely seen lesions following routine radiographic projections should lead to additional projections as needed.

Stress X-Rays

Stress films of the ankle, with the stress performed by an experienced clinician, can be most helpful in determining the presence and extent of ligament damage and chondral pathology. The normal range of talar tilt within the ankle mortise varies from minimal to up to 20 degrees in normal subjects. There is overlap between abnormal ankles and normal ankles in the upper limits of this range, so comparison views of the uninvolved side are essential for full evaluation. Stress films can be performed with abduction and adduction stress, direct anterior and posterior stress (drawer stress), and stresses in plantar and dorsiflexion. A variety of ligamentous supporting structures can be evaluated using appropriate stress views, and at the present time one of the authors (JFG) considers prearthroscopic stress films essential in all cases when utilizing distraction (Figures 4-4 through 4-8).

Radioisotope Scanning

Radioisotope scanning using bone-seeking radioisotopes can be a very useful adjunct procedure in detecting radiographically occult lesions of the ankle and in evaluating metabolic activity of known lesions. A wide range of uptake responses can be detected in ankle lesions studied prior to arthroscopy (Figures 4-9 through 4-11). Minimal uptake, which is diffuse, is frequently seen with early arthritis in a preradiographic stage. Subtle osteochondral lesions with minimal involvement of subchondral bone frequently appears as a more localized area of somewhat increased uptake. Pure chondral lesions should not incite increased radiographic isotope deposition. Mechanical alterations in the subchondral bone, however, or shallow osteochondral fractures, can cause enough local repair to stimulate further increased radioisotope deposition.

Often lesions which are radiographically invisible can appear as areas of

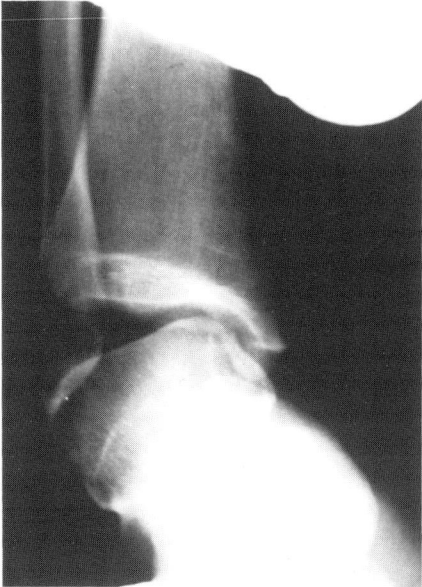

Figure 4-5. An AP x-ray of the right ankle shows marked angulation on varus stress. The patient had bilateral ankle pain following an automobile accident. Her ankle was arthroscoped by the referring orthopedic surgeon with no relief. While some instability was suspected, the author was surprised at the amount demonstrated by these preoperative studies.

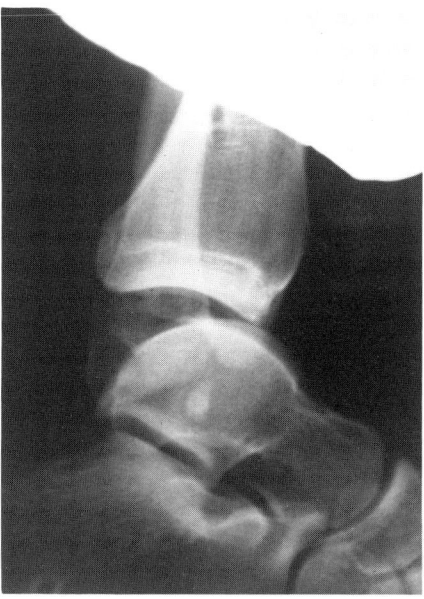

Figure 4-6. A lateral x-ray of the same ankle also shows marked anterior displacement.

Radiological Techniques 29

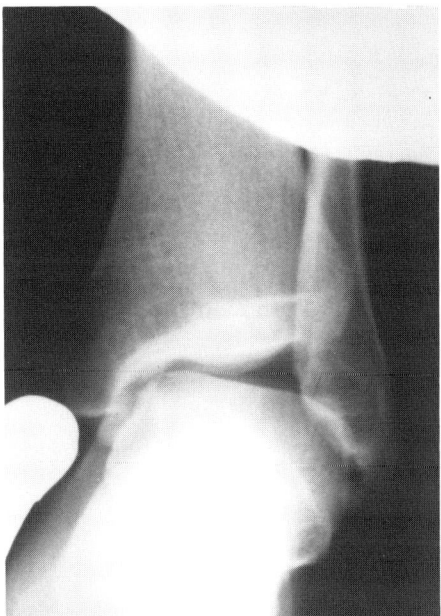

Figure 4-7. An AP x-ray of the same patient's left ankle shows less varus angulation.

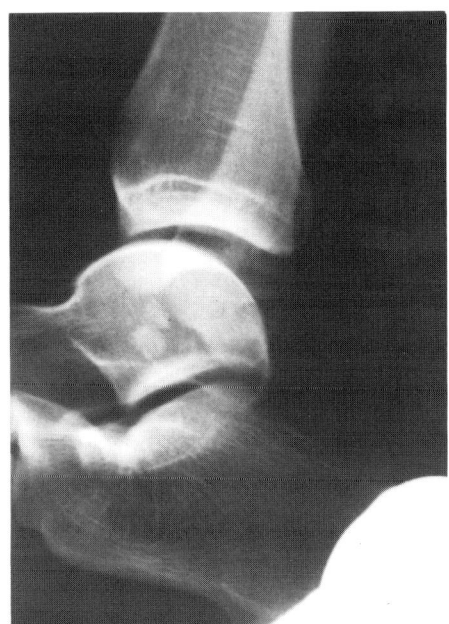

Figure 4-8. A lateral x-ray of the same ankle, when stressed anteriorly, again shows some anterior displacement, but also to a lesser degree. After further clinical evaluation, a lateral open tenodesis was done on the right ankle, which resulted in a marked improvement. Although it was felt that the left ankle could be normal (i.e., upper) for this patient, further history and progress seem to indicate otherwise. If further instability appears to be of clinical significance, in time, an arthroscopic ligamentous-capsular stapling will be considered by the author. This example shows the value of preoperative stress x-ray studies and the value of doing both ankles for comparison if it is felt to be indicated or in question.

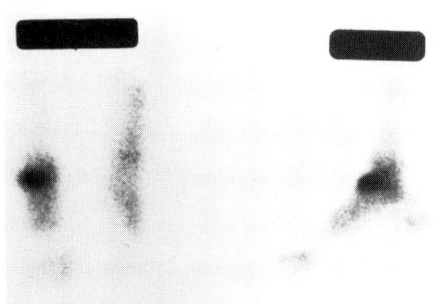

Figure 4-9. A bone scan shows marked concentration of radioisotopes in a lesion of osteochondritis dissecans.

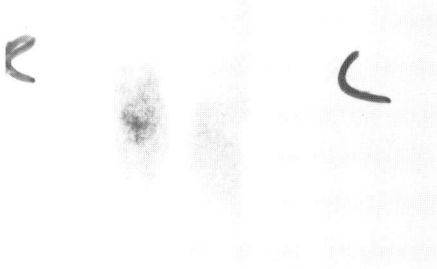

Figure 4-10. A bone scan demonstrates moderate increased uptake in the right ankle. An average sized osteocartilagenous lesion was seen on repeat standard x-ray views.

increased uptake on bone scans. Focal areas of increased uptake, ranging from moderate to intense, can be seen with most osteochondral lesions that are radiographically apparent. When used as a screening examination, a positive radioisotope scan can indicate a lesion requiring further anatomic evaluation. Diffuse uptake in the ankle may also signal the possibility of infection, which may require further evaluation with both radiologic techniques and specialized bone scanning examinations. Scanning with gallium 67 citrate or indium-labeled white cells may be helpful in evaluating the presence of infection.

Any bone scan performed for articular abnormality should include an immediate flow scan, a 20-minute postinjection scan to view the blood pool, and delayed views (three hours) to assess bone uptake of the isotope. Flow studies and blood-pool images can be extremely important in detecting localized soft tissue abnormality. Improved discrimination regarding focal bony lesions can be obtained by using single photon emission computed tomography in the adult, or pin-hole collimator images in children.

Conventional Tomography

Conventional tomography is helpful in defining the precise anatomic limits of a lesion detected on conventional x-rays. Conventional tomograms suffer from increased artifact and decreased resolution when compared to conventional x-rays, but can be effective when a lesion is obscured by overlying bone. For best discrimination of subtle lesions involving thin bones, such as the subchondral plate of the talus or tibial plafond, pleuridirectional tomograms with a 2mm to 5mm slice thickness should be obtained through the ankle in both anterior-posterior and lateral projections. The tomographic sections should be contiguous, and the kilovoltage should be low enough (80 Kvp or less) to allow adequate contrast. Arthrotomography following injection of contrast material into the ankle may have improved discrimination of

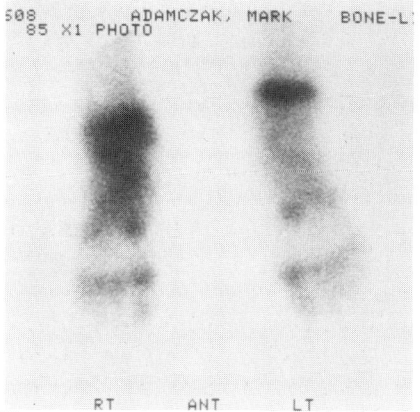

Figure 4-11. This bone scan showed marked, diffusely increased uptake in a 15-year-old boy with a low grade septic joint (See Chapter IX).

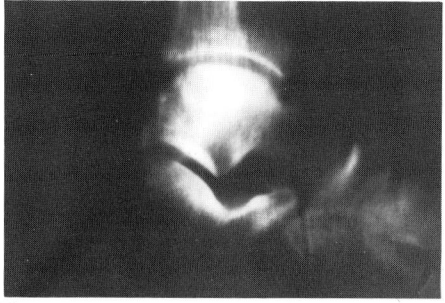

Figure 4-12. A lateral tomogram shows a large cyst in the posterior (lateral) talus.

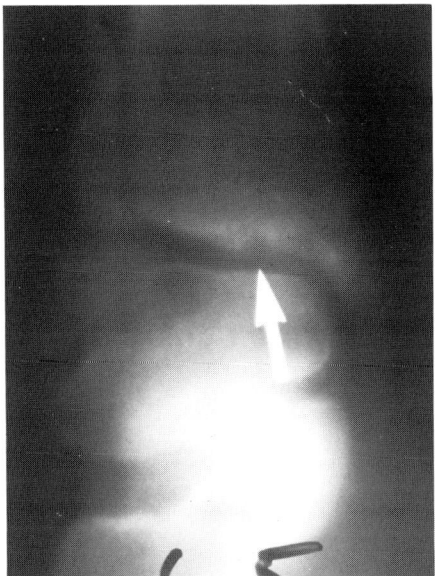

Figure 4-13. This AP tomogram shows a defect of the tibial plafond with a sclerotic base. This was not appreciated on routine films.

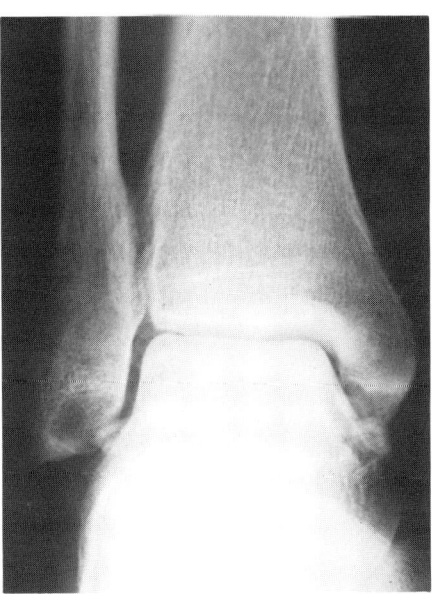

Figure 4-14. An AP x-ray in a symptomatic ankle shows suspected loose bodies.

subtle osteochondral lesions when compared to conventional tomograms (Figure 4-12). Examination in both radiographic projections is important, since the size (the anterior-posterior extent and the medial-lateral position) requires evaluation in two planes (Figure 4-13).

Arthrography

The major use of arthrography in ankle disorders is for evaluating the integrity of the ankle ligaments. On occasion, arthrograms, particularly arthrotomograms, can be helpful in evaluating osteochondral pathology and synovial surface abnormalities. Localized areas of cartilage thinning or chondral defects can be demonstrated arthrographically, and noncalcified intraarticular loose bodies can be detected using single-or double-contrast arthrograms or arthrotomography.

On occasion, the anterior impingement syndrome can be caused by intraarticular loose bodies. These loose bodies may be free or may be adherent to the synovium. Several examples of these lesions can be seen in this chapter and elsewhere in the text (Figures 4-14 through 4-19).

Arthrography can also be helpful in evaluating extraarticular calcifications thought to represent loose bodies radiographically. Sometimes arthrography can prove that a juxtaarticular calcification is, in fact, not a loose body but buried in the soft tissues and of no clinical significance. Synovial chondromatosis, as well as other localized capsular abnormalities, can be more readily diagnosed using arthrography (Figures 4-20 and 4-21) than conventional examinations. Many lesions in synovial (osteochondromatosis)

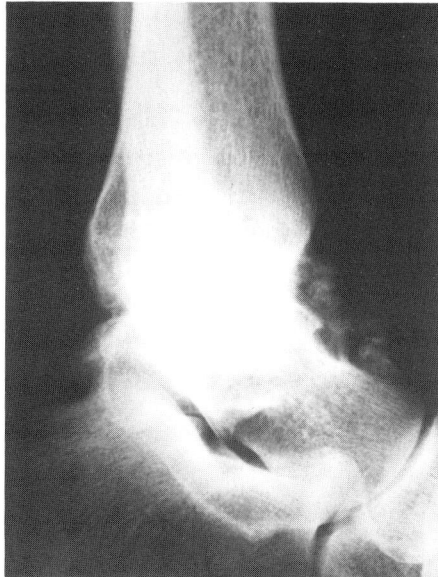

Figure 4-15. This lateral x-ray of the same patient shows anterior impingement symptoms. There was uncertainty whether these lesions were detached or fixed to the anterior synovium and capsule.

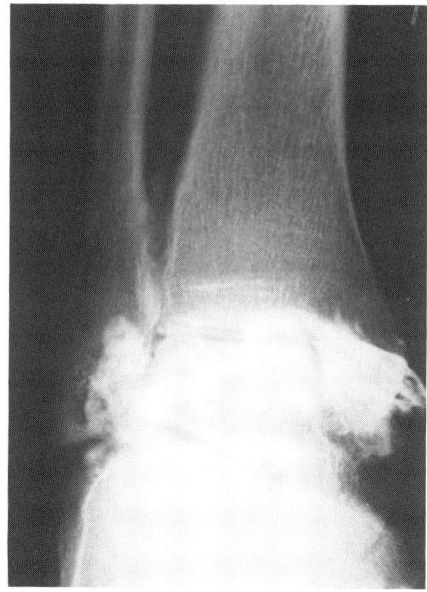

Figure 4-16. An AP arthrogram shows the loose bodies in the case cited above.

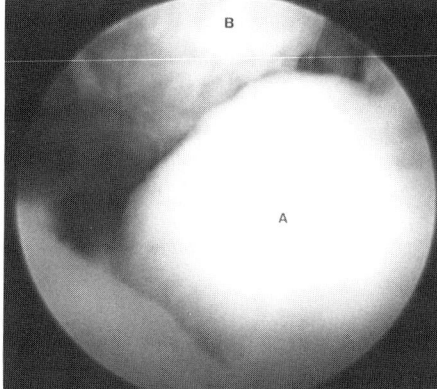

Figure 4-18. A large loose body (A) adjacent to the medial malleolus (B) and the anterior talus. Same case as above.

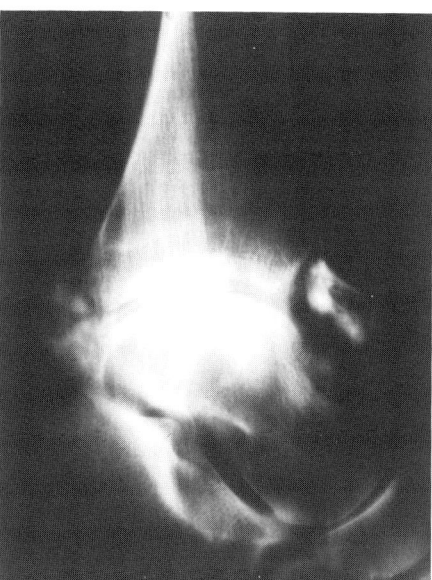

Figure 4-17. A lateral arthrotomogram in the same patient delineates the loose bodies in the anterior joint and shows at least one more in the posterior compartment.

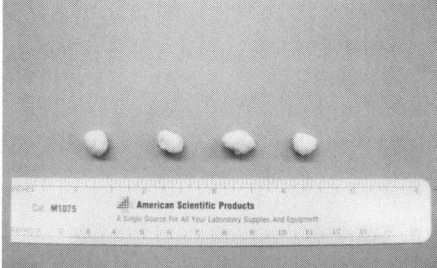

Figure 4-19. Shown are the four large loose bodies removed in the same case.

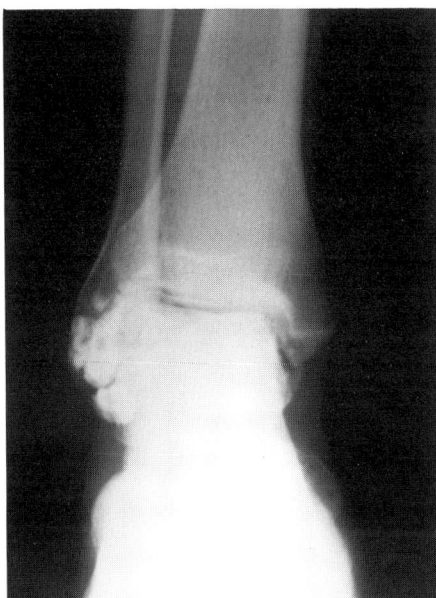 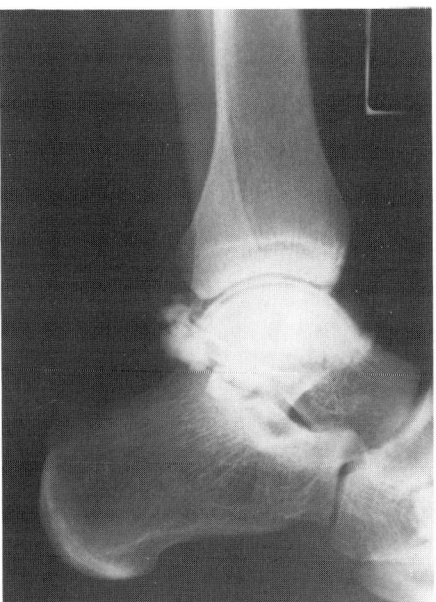

Figure 4-20. This is an AP arthrogram of synovial chondromatosis. Most lesions were in the posterolateral aspect of the ankle joint (See Chapter IX).

Figure 4-21. This lateral arthrogram shows the posterior lesions.

are not calcified. Calcified lesions can be readily seen on plain films, but arthrography may be necessary to determine the full extent of this disease. As with conventional films of the ankle, a full ankle series of views must be obtained to completely evaluate the joint.

Double-contrast or air-contrast arthrography can be particularly helpful in the postoperative patient. After reconstructive surgery of the talar dome, (excision, debridement, abrasion, and drilling), the extent of healing can be well shown using arthrography that can demonstrate that an osteochondral defect has "filled in" with fibrocartilage.

Other diffuse synovial disorders, such as inflammatory disease (rheumatoid arthritis, rheumatoid variant arthritis, etc.), pigmented villonodular synovitis, synovial ganglia, and adhesive or synechial capsulitis, are easily evaluated using arthrography. While the full range of arthrographic findings is beyond the scope of this chapter, detailed treatments of this subject are available in the radiologic literature. It must be emphasized that careful ankle arthrography can be an extremely useful method for evaluating the capsular surface in any case of unresolved clinical symptomatology in the ankle. Arthrography can be very useful and desirable prior to arthroscopy when evaluating the capsular surface and contour of the articular cartilage prior to direct inspection.

Computed Tomography

Computed tomography (CT) has largely replaced conventional tomogra-

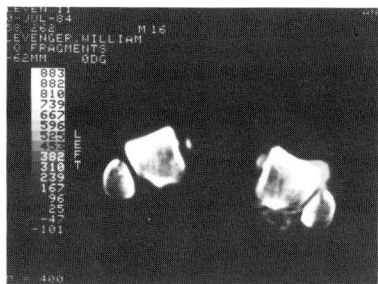

Figure 4-22. A CT scan shows chondral lesions in the left posterior ankle joint that were removed at arthroscopy. These were not seen on the other x-ray studies.

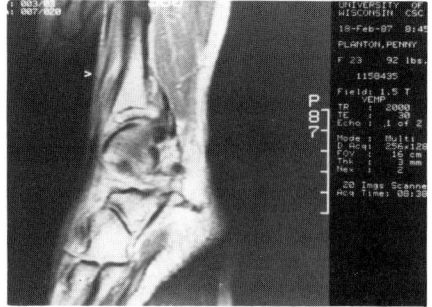

Figure 4-23. MR shows tendinitis of the extensor digitorum communis tendon (arrow). This patient had only temporary relief with the arthroscopic removal of a minimal synovial impingement lesion earlier. She returned to long distance running too soon and developed recurrent symptoms. Further open surgery was required to explore the tendon and gave relief.

phy in evaluating subtle lesions of the talar dome and tibial plafond. While CT cannot discriminate soft tissues well, and is therefore predominantly useful for bone lesions, the unparalleled ability of CT to produce tomographic images free of overlying artifacts makes it a major contributor to evaluating the talar dome (Figure 4-22). The radiation dose in computed tomography is essentially the same in the ankles as that received during conventional tomography, but the scatter radiation to the patient is considerably less. Modern CT scanners have a large enough gantry to allow direct coronal imaging, probably the most useful CT projection. In most cases today computed tomography has supplanted conventional tomography as the procedure of choice when a tomographic procedure is necessary.

Magnetic Resonance Imaging

Magnetic resonance imaging is in its infancy, and its exact role in evaluating articular abnormality has not been defined. No ionizing radiation is used for MR, and images are produced in essentially any anatomic plane without the need for reformatting (a technique which can degrade CT images). While there are a multitude of technical factors under evaluation to decide which MR technique will be best for evaluating joints, some statements can be made concerning its usefulness today.

MR offers unparalleled resolution of soft tissue structures, including fat pads, tendons, and capsular surfaces (Figure 4-23). The ability of MR to produce images in a variety of projections on occasion leads to diagnosis of bony lesions that can be too subtle for radiographic techniques. This may be particularly useful in cases with positive radioisotope scans but negative radiographic studies (Figures 4-24 through 4-27). It is practically certain that specialized surface coils will be needed to evaluate any joint, and the ankle is

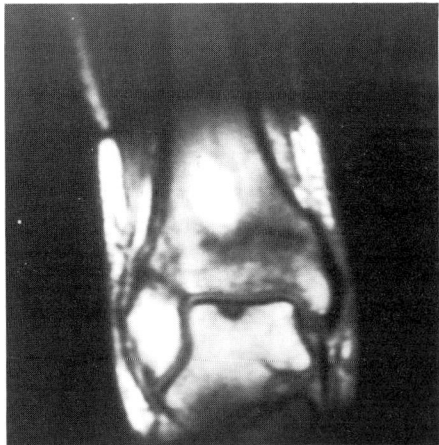

Figure 4-24. This AP MR shows a large, central osteocartilagenous defect of the central talus not seen on routine films or tomograms in both planes.

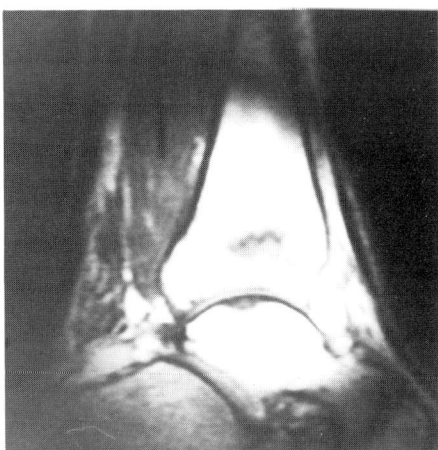

Figure 4-25. An MR lateral view of the above. The articular cartilage was intact at arthroscopy.

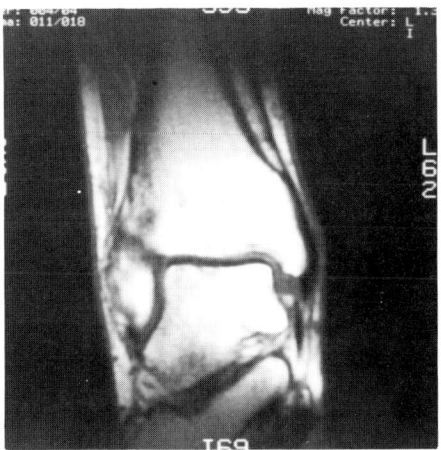

Figure 4-26. An AP MR at 2 months postoperatively. The lesion was drilled with fine (.062) Kirschner wires during an arthroscopy, utilizing the transmalleolar approach. The arthroscopic anterior cruciate ligament guide was used for accuracy in wire placement.

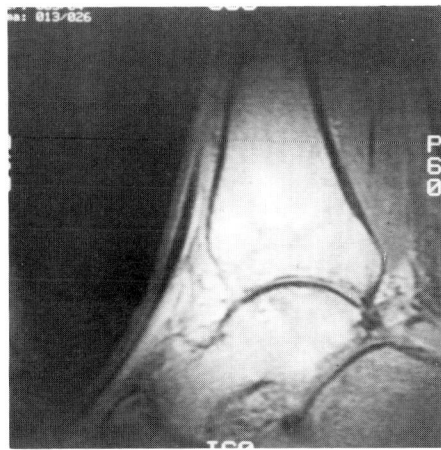

Figure 4-27. This lateral MR also demonstrates healing.

no exception. Some investigators have reported that a variety of lesions produce characteristic MR appearances that they have found useful in evaluating a variety of abnormalities. It must be emphasized, however, that these findings are highly preliminary and are not as yet accepted throughout the radiologic community. Much further research needs to be done with this exciting modality to define its role in evaluating the ankle prior to arthroscopy.

Motion-Record Studies

The full evaluation of the presence and mobility of intraarticular lesions, such as loose bodies, can be very important prior to arthroscopy. Static techniques, such as conventional films, arthrograms, and tomograms, can be somewhat confusing when reviewed prior to arthroscopy. In the past, cineradiography was used to document the fluoroscopic findings prior to arthrography, in an effort to document the size, number, and motion of various intraarticular lesions. Today, the use of online videotape has essentially replaced cineradiography, and should be considered an important addition to arthrographic or fluoroscopic examination of the ankle in documenting the dynamic abnormalities within the ankle.

Xeroradiography

Xeroradiography has been used in the past to evaluate the soft tissues. Extensive use for xeroradiography in mammography has proven its usefulness in discriminating soft tissue lesions and microcalcifications. There is decreasing use and availability of xeroradiography today, with new film screen combinations available to evaluate the soft tissues. The future role of xeroradiography, particularly if CT or MR is available, is uncertain.

Conclusion

Full radiographic examination of the disordered ankle is essential prior to arthroscopy. At the least a good conventional x-ray examination is necessary to evaluate gross bony anatomy and subtle bony lesions. Tomographic techniques, such as CT or, on occasion, conventional arthrography or arthrotomography, can resolve a subtle radiographic abnormality. Radioisotope scanning is useful in detecting radiographically visible occult lesions or to screen for intraarticular pathology in the chronically painful ankle. If abnormalities are not resolved during conventional examination, more sophisticated modalities should be used until as complete an evaluation as possible has been obtained prior to arthroscopic study.

References
1. Smith GR, Winquist RA: Subtle Transchondral Fractures of the Talar Dome: A Radiological Perspective. Rad 124: 667-673, 1977.
2. Dalinka MK: Arthrography. New York, Springer-Verlage, 1980.

CHAPTER 5

INSTRUMENTATION IN ARTHROSCOPIC SURGERY OF THE ANKLE

J. Serge Parisien, M.D.

At the present time arthroscopy of the ankle is a well-established procedure in the evaluation and management of some ankle disorders. The technique is demanding, and a successful approach requires a good knowledge of the regional anatomy and familiarity with the arthroscopic portals. Operative arthroscopy of the ankle is, for all practical purposes, excisional in nature. Up to approximately one year ago, most surgical procedures performed on the ankle used surgical tools borrowed from knee surgical instrument sets (Figures 5-1 through 5-5).[6] More recently, some specialized instrumentation systems were made available in order to solve problems specific to the ankle joint. Shorter and smaller arthroscopes with better optics for joint visualization, lighter cameras, shorter hand instruments and smaller power instrumentation, distracting devices, and ankle holders make the task of the arthroscopic surgeon much easier.

This chapter is intended to be an overview of the surgical instrumentation useful in arthroscopic surgery of the ankle. This list, however, is not exhaustive, and although some surgical instruments are listed by name, comparable instruments are offered by many other manufacturers. For purposes of clarity, instrumentation for diagnostic and operative arthroscopy of the ankle can be classified into the following categories: instruments for viewing, excisional instruments, instruments for reconstruction, retrieving instruments, and accessory instruments.

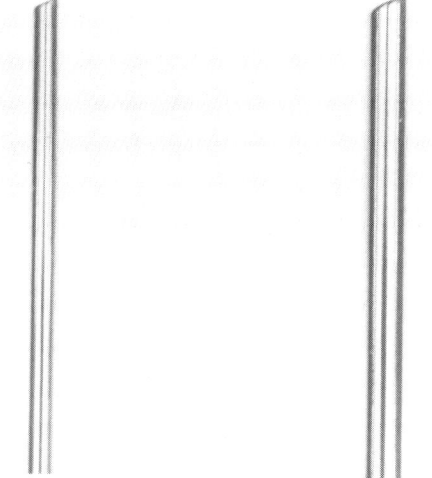

Figure 5-1. 25 degree arthroscopes, 2.7mm and 4mm.

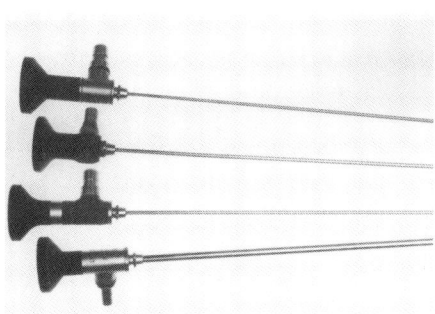

Figure 5-2. 10 to 25 degree arthroscopes with different angulations, 2.2mm, 2.7mm, and 4mm.

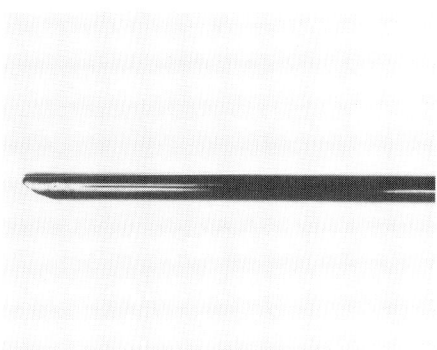

Figure 5-3A. 70 degree angled arthroscope, 4mm.

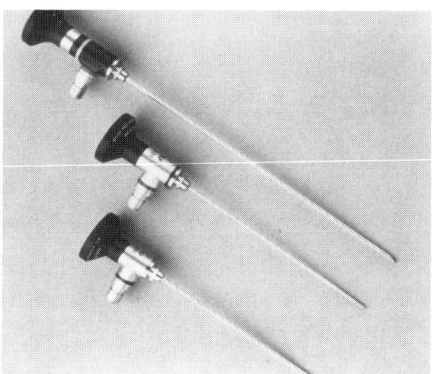

Figure 5-3B. Small joint arthroscopy set with regular 2.7mm and shorter 2.2mm and 2.7mm scopes.

Instruments for Viewing

Arthroscopes and Light Cables

It is not our purpose to review the different types of arthroscopes. The reader is referred to some excellent articles in the literature for more information on this subject.[7,8] Suffice it to say that most arthroscopes used at the present time are of the rod lens type system, originally designed by Professor Hopkins of England. In this system, glass cylinders are separated by relatively small air spaces.

Arthroscopes, varying in size from 2.2mm to 2.9mm, were originally designed for visualization of small joints. Larger arthroscopes, such as the 4mm that allows continuous flow through the arthroscope sheath, were preferred by some surgeons since they were thought to deliver a better image when used with a video camera. However, shorter and smaller size arthroscopes are now available with comparable brightness and quality image transmission.

Arthroscopes with angulation of view of 30 degrees are most suitable for visualization of the ankle joint. The 70 degree inclined view can also be helpful in some situations, and, with some practice, orientation with this type of arthroscope may be easier (Figures 5-1 through 5-3). Many high intensity light sources are available for performance of arthroscopic surgery with the television camera. Light cables with different adapters for various arthroscopes or light sources are important for transmission of light. They are usually two basic types: the bundle light cables and the liquid light guides. Although the liquid light guides transmit considerably more light than the bundle light cables, they are not flexible and are difficult to manipulate.

Video Cameras

The video cameras usually are of two types: the tube and solid state.[9] The video tube camera weighs from 6oz to 8oz, and, since it is not soakable, it requires the use of plastic sterile covers for draping. The second type of camera, the solid state video camera, is much lighter and can be soaked in glutaraldehyde. Its lighter size also allows easy manipulation of the arthroscope for a joint such as the ankle (Figure 5-4).

Inflow Systems

At the beginning of the diagnostic part of the procedure, a 60cc syringe and a small plastic tubing are useful for continuous irrigation of the joint. To obtain sufficient hydrostatic pressure and continuous flow for distention of the joint during arthroscopic surgery, plastic bag containers capable of holding six liters of fluid, either normal saline or Ringer's lactate, are usually placed above the patient on a well-secured IV pole. Small cannulas and small adapters for the plastic tubing are useful (Figures 5-5 and 5-6). The cannulas can be used either for inflow or outflow during arthroscopic surgery. When they are used as outflow cannulas, the inflow system is attached to the sheath of the arthroscope. Some surgeons use them for the inflow system, and, in that situation, the outflow is attached directly to the arthroscope.

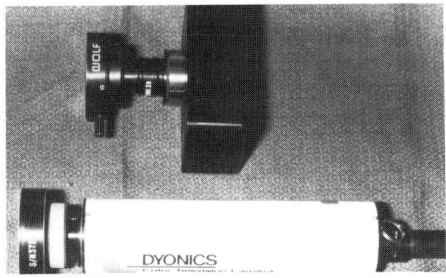

Figure 5-4. Solid state video camera and tube camera.

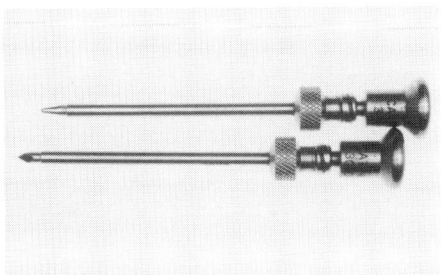

Figure 5-5. Small cannulas with smooth and sharp obturators (Dyonics).

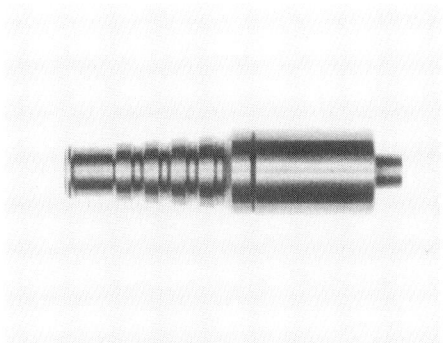

Figure 5-6. Adaptor for small cannula.

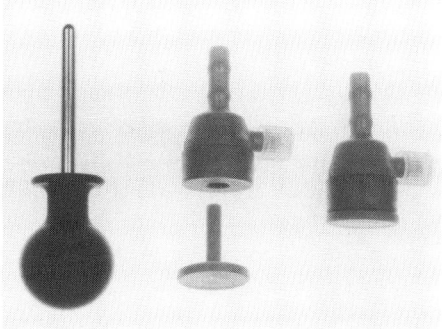

Figure 5-7. Small disposable cannula system (Acufex).

Disposable Arthroscopic Cannulas

A disposable cannula system is available for arthroscopic surgery of the ankle (Figure 5-7). The benefits of the system are numerous. The presence of a double seal will prevent leaking of the fluid medium. The side port allows inflow or outflow of saline or Ringer lactate, eliminating the need for an accessory portal. The soft tissue is also protected when inserting and removing the surgical instruments.

Excisional Instruments

These instruments can be subdivided into hand instruments and motorized instruments.

Hand instruments.

Spinal Needles 18-gauge needles are commonly used during arthroscopic surgery of the ankle for distention of the capsule prior to the introduction of the arthroscope and for careful palpation of the intra-articular structures (Figure 5-8). They also allow precise positioning of the arthroscopic portal before the placement of the skin incision.

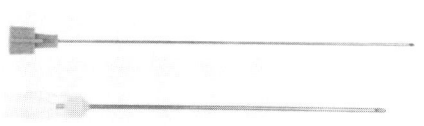

Figure 5-8. 18-gauge spinal needle.

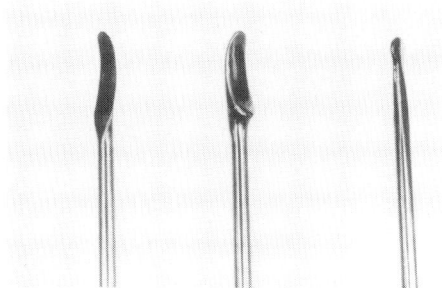

Figure 5-9. Different instruments that can be used for probing (Acufex).

Small Probes. Probes 1mm in size can be used in the ankle joint for palpation and manipulation of articular cartilage defects or loose bodies. A flat-ended probe that can be introduced through the disposable plastic cannula is also available. Aside from the ease of insertion, this probe can eliminate damage to the articular cartilage. A specially contoured probe can also be used for palpation and manipulation of osteochondral defects or softer areas of articular cartilage of the talar dome or tibial plafond (Figure 5-9).

Cutting Instruments. The small confines of the ankle joint have resulted in the development of special blades. These blades are sharp, resistant, and have magnetic properties. They are shorter and can be delivered into the joint through the disposable cannula system. One blade has cutting edges on both sides and, although semipointed, is not sharp at the tip. The curvature of the blade permits gradual insertion into the base of the intra-articular defect or soft area of the articular cartilage. Some blades have a cutting edge on one side to protect adjacent tissue during the manipulation into the joint. These knives can be used for sectioning fibrous bands, plicae, and capsular tissue (Figures 5-10 and 5-11).

Basket Forceps. Small straight basket forceps can be used as cutting instruments during arthroscopic surgery of the ankle. They can be useful in performing initial debridement of tough fibrous tissue and soft articular areas on the anterior aspect of the tibial plafond.

Small Size Scissors. Small scissors that are sharp enough to grasp and cut fibrous bands in the anterior or posterior compartment of the ankle joint can be of great help during arthroscopic surgery of the ankle. Small sharp curettes are particularly useful in trimming the edges or excising fibrous tissue from the surface of an osteochondral defect (Figure 5-12).

Small Rasps. Small rasps are used to contour the joint surface after excision of an osteophyte or for abrasion of exposed cortical bone (Figure 5-13).

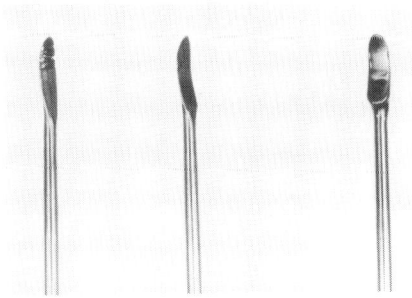

Figure 5-10. Different types of knives for surgical arthroscopy of the ankle (Acufex).

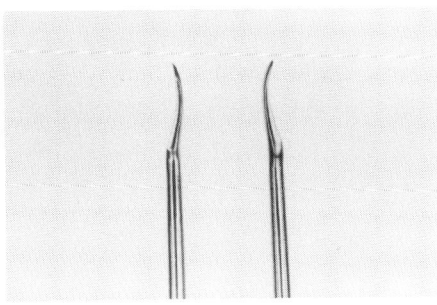

Figure 5-11. Blades with cutting edge on one side (Acufex).

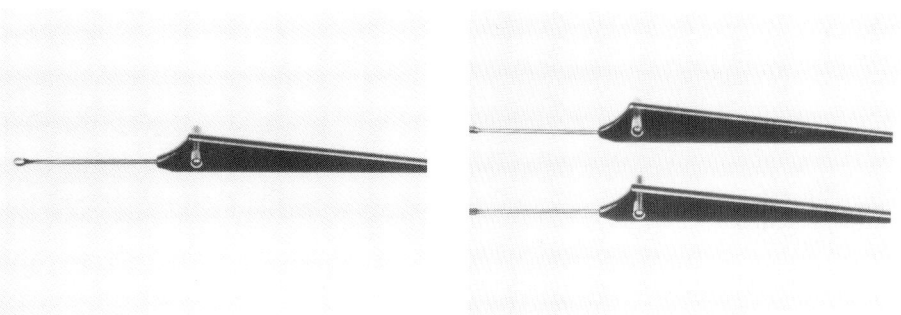

Figure 5-12. Small curette (Acufex).

Figure 5-13. Different shapes of rasps (Acufex).

Small Grasping Forceps. These can be passed through the disposable plastic cannula system are available for grasping small osteochondral bodies. The jaws have teeth that reduce the chances of slipping of the loose body.

Pituitary Forceps. Up and down biters of small size are particularly helpful in removing floating fragments from the lateral and medial recesses of the ankle joint. They can also be used to debride degenerated articular cartilage or scar tissue from the anterior aspect of the ankle (Figure 5-14).

Motorized Instrumentation

The Intra-articular Shaver System. This was developed by Lanny Johnson[10], and was originally used by us to perform debridement in ankle arthroscopy (Figure 5-15). However, when using the cutter head capable of excising tough fibrous adhesions and hypertrophic synovial tissue, damage to the articular cartilage can be done. At the present time, a miniature small joint system is available with a more powerful motor. It has more revolutions per minute than the first generation intra-articular shaver, and can be used quite well in joints such as the elbow, ankle, subtalar, and wrist. A small

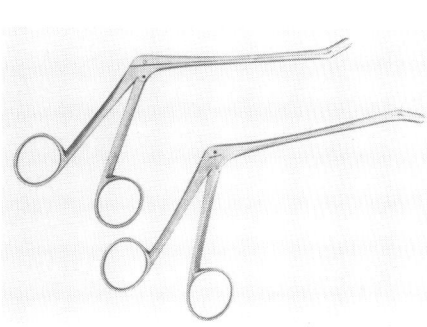

Figure 5-14. Pituitary forceps (Acufex).

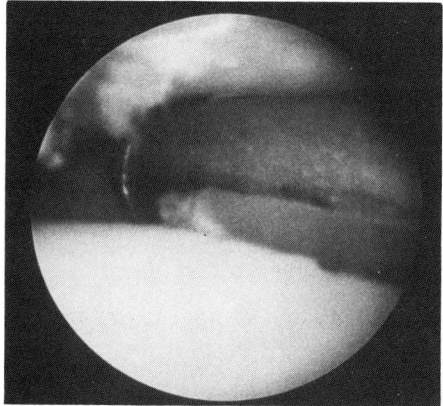

Figure 5-15. Small intra-articular shaver performing joint debridement.

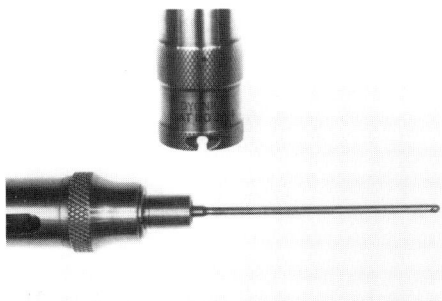
Figure 5-16. Small arthroplasty instrument.

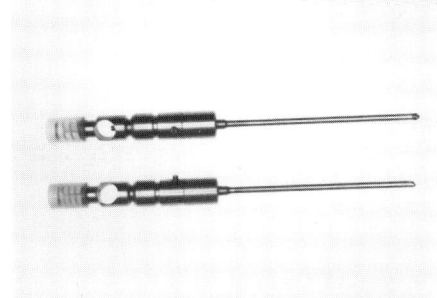
Figure 5-17. 2.8mm resector and abrader.

resector, as well as a small abrador 2.8mm in size, can be used for synovectomy and debridement of adhesions, arthroscopic resection of osteophytes, and abrasion of exposed cortical surfaces (Figures 5-16 through 5-20). Small solid shaft drill bits can be used for drilling of osteochondral defects or stable osteochondral lesions of the talar dome. Cannulated drill bits can also be used over Kirschner wires through a transmalleolar approach for drilling of posterior lesions of the talus.

Instrumentation for Repair

An arthroscopic instrumentation for ligamentous and capsular repair is available (Instrument Makar) at the present time. Originally designed for reattachment of torn anterior cruciate ligaments and repair of glenohumeral ligaments, its use has been extended to the ankle joint[11] for the arthroscopic reconstruction of chronic lateral instability. A cannula with its obturator, a driver-extractor, and staples with reverse-angle teeth of two different sizes (5.5mm and 6.7mm) are part of the instrumentation (Figure 5-21). Small size staples are used for the ankle, and the technique is described in detail in Chapter XI.

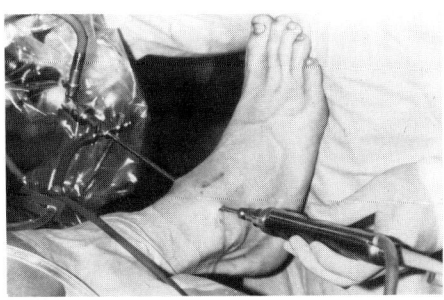
Figure 5-18. Small arthroplasty system through anterolateral portal and 4mm arthroscope through anteromedial portal.

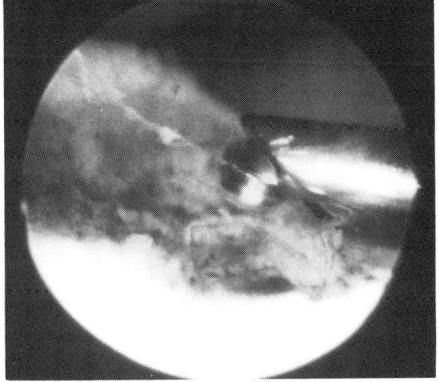
Figure 5-19. Abrader performing abrasion of osteochondral defect, anterolateral aspect of left ankle.

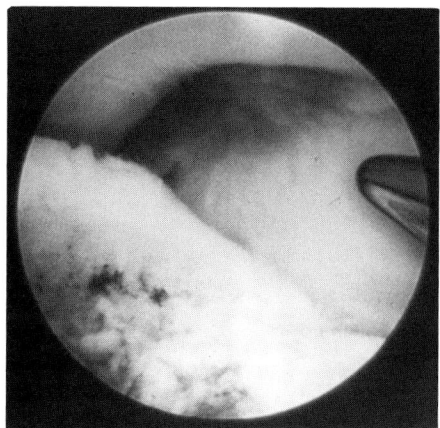 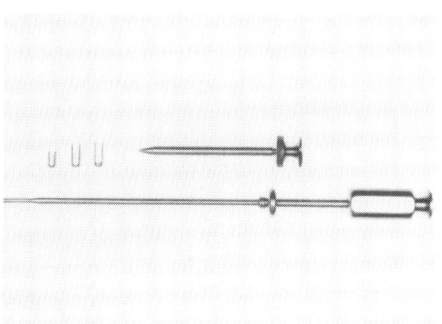

Figure 5-20. Probe palpating articular cartilage of lateral malleolus osteochondral defect, left side of picture.

Figure 5-21. Instrumentation for ligamentous repair (Instrument Makar).

Retrieving Instruments

Metallic tubes with suction and magnetic properties on one end have been effective in immobilizing and retrieving broken instrument fragments during arthroscopic surgery. With a large fragment, after mobilization to a more accessible and superficial position for retrieval a small arthrotomy incision sometimes is mandatory to remove the fragment (Figure 5-22).

Accessory Instruments

Ankle Holder (Acufex)

Recently, an ankle holder was developed for use in arthroscopy of the ankle. This holder is totally autoclavable and can be fitted into a standard Clark clamp. The foot platform has a ball joint with a clamp lock that allows adjustment in three axes. Since the knee has to be flexed, the ankle holder is usually used in conjunction with a leg holder that is raised above the table. In a more recent design, the cushions of the bean bag can be rotated to any desired position, thus facilitating the plantar position of the foot (Figure 5-23).

Aiming Device (Acufex)

Many jigs have been developed for arthroscopic anterior cruciate reconstruction that allow the precise insertion of intra-articualr wires from a point outside the joint. These devices can be used in the ankle joint for accurate placement of guide wires or cannulated reamers, through transmalleolar portals for drilling or curettage of some posteriorly located lesions of the talar dome. This technique is described in detail elsewhere in the book.

Mechanical Distractor (Acufex)

Tightness of some ankle joints not only makes visualization of the intra-

Figure 5-22. Retrieving instruments (Acufex).

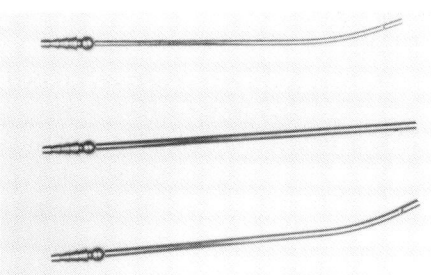

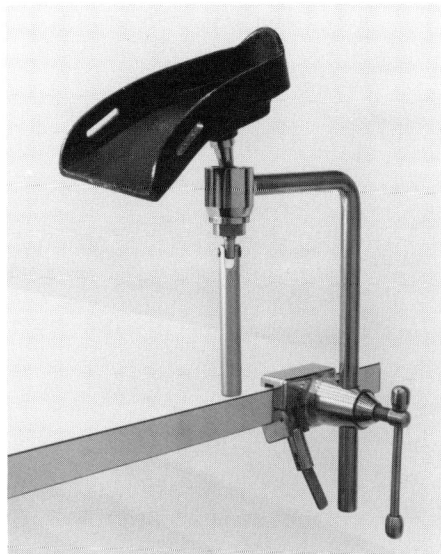

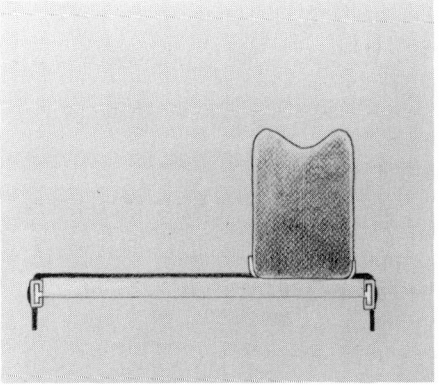

Figure 5-23A. Ankle holder showing foot platform and clamp lock (Acufex).

Figure 5-23B. Leg holder that can be used in conjunction with the inflatable bean bag (Acufex).

articular structures challenging, but also makes the manipulation of surgical instruments difficult and at times hazardous, and the risks of scuffing the articular cartilage and breaking surgical instruments are potentially increased. Using external fixator apparatus, we have successfully performed in the past some distraction of the joint with improved visualization and ease of manipulation of instruments. However, the pins would transfix the tibia and os calcis and would allow motion in one plane only. A mechanical distractor is at the present time available for use. This apparatus can be placed on either side of the ankle with pins not requiring complete inversion into the bones. A ball joint placed at the distal part makes dorsiflexion and plantarflexion possible, as well as varus or valgus position of the foot. (Figures 5-24 and 5-25).

Arthroscopy Pump

A device allowing a reliable way to control independently pressure and flow inside the joint during the performance of arthroscopic surgery is available. By increasing the flow, the field of view can be cleared easily of blood and articular debris. If better distention of the joint is needed, the pressure can be increased wihout affecting the flow. Pressure control from 0mm to 18mm Hg and flow control from 0ml to 975ml per minute can be obtained (Figure 5-26).

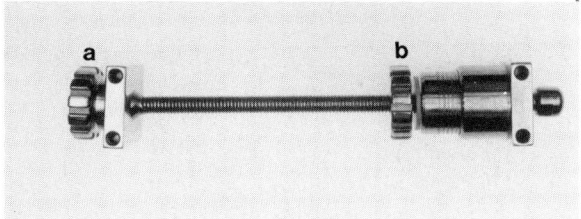

Figure 5-24. Mechanical distractor (Acufex). (a) Knob to tighten universal joint at distal part of distractor; (b) Knob for distraction.

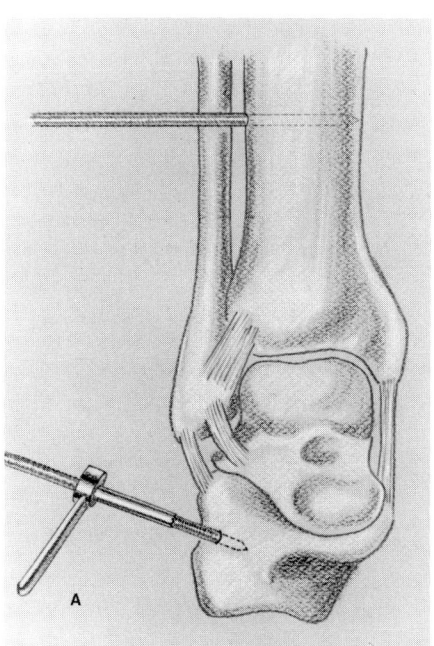
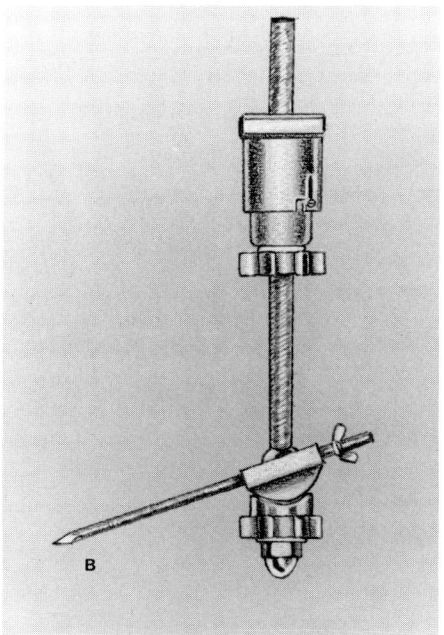

Figure 5-25. Ball joint at distal part of distractor allows different positions of the foot while ankle is distracted. Strain gauge is used for reference. A) Pin inserted at 20° downward inclination through os calcis becomes parallel with proximal pin when ankle is distracted. B) Note strain gauge and wing nut.

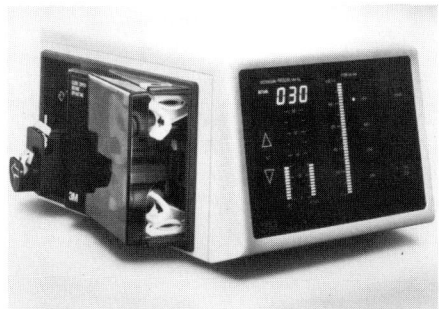

Figure 5-26. Arthroscopy pump that can be used for arthroscopy of the ankle (3-M).

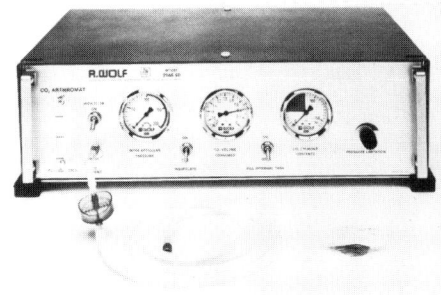

Figure 5-27. Insufflator for arthroscopy in gas medium (Wolf).

Insufflator for Arthroscopic Surgery in Gas Medium

Bircher was the first one to use a mixture of oxygen and nitrogen for examination of the knee joint.[12] The technique was popularized by Henche, who advocated the use of CO_2 as a medium for arthroscopy of the knee.[13] A special unit called Arthro-pneu gives pressure between 50mm and 80mm Hg. Ericksson has reported the use of gas arthroscopy in joints such as the elbow, hip, and ankle, and claims that gas arthroscopy, by pressing away the synovial folds, allows better inspection of the joint.[14] Apparently, also the field of vision of any optical system is larger in gas than in fluid. Because of the possibility of CO_2 causing irritation of the joint and dilation of the blood vessels, Ericksson[14] has advocated the use of dry air with bacterial filter. In his experience, there have been no complications. Some problems are, however, associated with the use of gas, such as occasional clouding of the lens and escaping of gas, requiring the use of small incisions (Figure 5-27).

Summary

Arthroscopy is a valuable tool in the diagnosis and treatment of ankle pathology. The recent introduction of some new equipment makes the procedure easier, even in tight joints. Arthroscopic instruments are not only delicate, but expensive. Their durability and optimal use require delicate handling and proper care.[15] To achieve this goal, the role of the nurse in charge of instrumentation in any arthroscopy unit cannot be over-emphasized.

References

1. Drez D, Guhl JF, Gollehon DL: Ankle Arthroscopy Technique and Indications. J Foot & Ankle 2:138-143, 1981.
2. Guhl JF: New Techniques for Arthroscopic Surgery of the Ankle: Preliminary Report. Orth 9:260-269, 1986.
3. Parisien JS and Shereff MJ: The Role of Arthroscopy in the Diagnosis and Management of Disorders of the Ankle. J Foot & Ankle, 2(3): 144-149, 1981.
4. Parisien JS: The Role of Arthroscopy in the Treatment of Transchondral

Fractures of the Talus. Am J of Sports Med 14: 210-217, 1986.
5. Baker CL, Andrews JR, Ryan JB: Arthroscopic Treatment of Transchondral Talar Dome Fractures — Arthroscopy. J of Arthroscopic & Related Surg 2: 82-87, 1986.
6. Parisien JS: Diagnostic and Operative Arthroscopy of the Ankle: Technique and Indications. Bul Hospital for Joint Diseases 45: 38-47, 1985.
7. Prescott R: Optical Design and Care of the Endoscope, in AAOS, Symposium on Arthroscopy and Arthrography of the Knee. St. Louis, Mosby, 1978, 13-25.
8. Berci G: Endoscopy. New York, Appleton-Century Crofts, 1976.
9. Jackson DW, Gvadia DN: Video-Arthroscopy: Present and Future Developments. J of Arthroscopic & Related Surg 2: 108-115, 1985.
10. Johnson L: Use of Cartilage Shaver. Los Angeles, 1978.
11. Hawkins RB: Arthroscopic Reconstruction for Chronic Lateral Instability of the Ankle in Arthroscopic Surgery Update. McGinty J, ed. Rockville, Aspen, 1985, 175-181.
12. Bircher E: Die Arthroendoskopie. Zbl Chir 48:1460-1461, 1921.
13. Henche HR: Arthroscopy of the Knee Joint. New York, Springer-Verlag, 1979.
14. Eriksson E, Sebik A: Arthroscopy and Arthroscopic Surgery in a Gas Versus a Fluid Medium. Orthop Clin North America 13: 293-298, 1982.
15. Cable AM: The Care of Arthroscopic Equipment in Arthroscopic Surgery Update. McGinty J, ed. Rockville, Aspen, 1985, 13-20.

CHAPTER 6

PORTALS AND TECHNIQUES

James F. Guhl, M.D.

The techniques recently introduced for arthroscopy and arthroscopic surgery of the ankle will be described in this portion of the text. The proper positioning of the patient to gain optimum access to this joint is essential. The operating room setup and the relationship of the team is as important, if not more so, as it is in arthroscopic surgery of the knee, shoulder, and elbow. The utilization of the available approaches will be shown with combinations for triangulating and performing surgery. The key to these techniques is mechanical distraction of the joint, and the employment of the ankle holder.

Mechanical distraction between the tibia and talus is utilized, along with the transmalleolar approaches (illustrated later), for treating talar dome defects. This combined with the ankle holder and improved development of the posterolateral approach allows the surgeon to carry out a complete procedure for treatment of all pathology encountered in the ankle.

Operating instruments for arthroscopic surgery of the ankle have been recently designed and are commercially available (See Chapter V). These, along with the above innovations, will further add to the development of arthroscopic surgery of this joint.

The distraction method is carried out by placing a threaded pin through the lower tibia and the os calcis. The distractor then gradually separates the articular surface of the tibial plafond and talar dome to a distance of about 7mm to 8mm. The advantages of distraction are: increased room for viewing with elimination of blind spots, especially in the mid-and posterior compartments. There is more room to triangulate and manipulate instruments in all of these areas. Chondral defects can be evaluated and more thoroughly probed. Lesions that were previously not accessible can be seen and treated arthroscopically. Loose bodies will be retrieved with greater assurance, and a more complete synovectomy is now possible.

Some early cases of fibroarthrosis and capsulitis can be treated with distraction and manipulation. There is also improved correlation with x-ray techniques, since the ankle joint is now more thoroughly understood. As this method was employed, the author noted that scuffing was reduced considerably. There is less fluid extravasation around the ankle and into the compartments of the leg. This is because the ankle joint is easier to enter and therefore to maintain the portals, while infusinq saline. The possibility of instrument breakage has also been significantly reduced with more space to work. Performance of arthroscopic ankle surgery therefore was found to be much less demanding and there was less reliance on an assistant for maintaining distraction. Furthermore, preoperative clinical evaluation, as illustrated in this text, along with properly selected x-ray techniques, will result in a higher percentage of pathological findings than when performing arthroscopy of the knee and shoulder joints.

The disadvantages of distraction are the potential complications, such as broken pins, and pin tract problems. Damage to neurovascular and anatomical structures is possible. The pin holes in the tibia and os calcis are potential stress risers and could lead to a fracture. However, these problems should not occur, unless the distraction method is not properly executed. Ligament stretching or disruption, as discussed, should not be a cause of concern.

Operating Room Setup and Positioning

Ankle arthroscopy is done under general or spinal anesthesia in a standard hospital operating room, or a freestanding surgical center. The setup, including the placement of the team, video monitors and equipment, is important for efficiency. Selected x-rays are placed on display for reference.

The patient is placed in the supine position on the operating room table. A sandbag is placed under the buttocks, on the involved side, to maintain a vertical position of the ankle and foot and avoid external rotation of the extremity. The ankle is placed as close to the end of the table as possible for easy access while performing surgery. The bean bag is employed and elevated about 12 to 14 inches above the level of the operating table with the aid of a special post. Most knee holders can be adapted for this purpose. This allows more acute flexion of the hip and knee, placing the ankle and foot plantigrade when attached to the ankle holder. A tourniquet applied at the time of surgery is inflated at 300mm to 350mm of mercury (or about 100mm above systolic pressure), at the discretion of the surgeon. The ankle holder is sterile and clamped over the drapes to a bar at the end of the table. All drapes should be snug around the leg, thigh, and buttocks to allow room for manipulation of the instruments, arthroscope, and camera, when the need for the posterior portals is required. Ace bandages and Coban should be wrapped around the drapes for this purpose. Internal rotation of the foot and ankle allows easier entry of the arthroscope and instruments from posterolateral, since the buttocks, thigh, and operating table are then well out of the way. The ankle holder can be adjusted to further extend the extremity if necessary when surgery of the ankle joint is expected to be confined or shifted back to the anterior compartment (Figures 6-1 through 6-3).

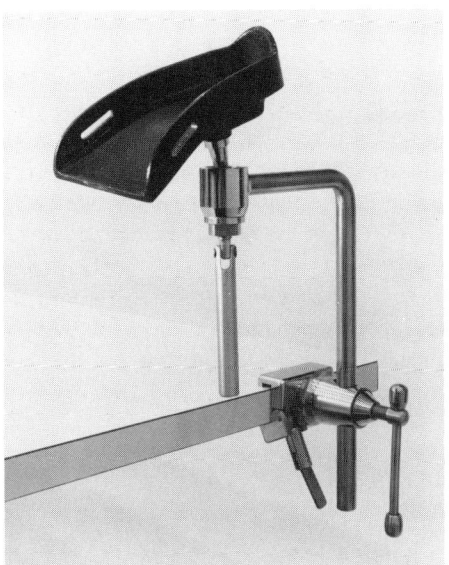

Figure 6-1. The ankle holder (Acufex).

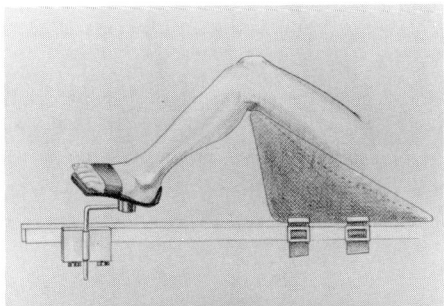

Figure 6-2. Bean bag supporting thigh with acutely flexed hip and knee (Acufex). This allows foot and ankle to be held in relatively plantigrade position. Note that angle at apex of bean bag is 80°. Bean bag can be adjusted during inflation to comply with anatomy.

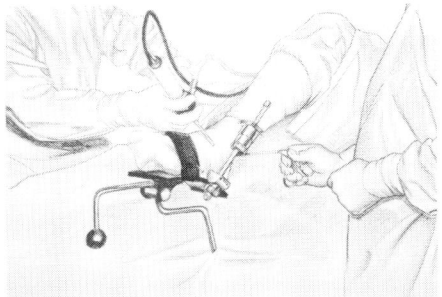

Figure 6-3. This is a view of the operating room setup for ankle arthroscopy. The patient's hip and knee are acutely flexed. Viewing through the arthroscope is done from the anterolateral portal, and a grasping forceps is inserted into the posterolateral portal. The reverse position of the arthroscope and instruments can be employed. Any one of the three anterior portals can be utilized.

Surgery can be performed with the patient supine and the knee flexed over any type of support to gain a similar position. However, with out the knee-ankle holder set up it is difficult to maintain control and there is not enough room to get behind the ankle for the posterior approach.

When prepping and draping have been completed, the anatomical structures are located and drawn on the skin with a marking pencil. Transillumination, or the placement of the light cable against the skin, will often show the superficial neurovascular structures.

Mechanical Distraction

The latest model of the distraction device used at the time of this writing is illustrated (Figure 6-4, Acufex). New features for safety and efficiency are elimination of a wrench system, the pivot action of the pin grip of the distal end to prevent pin bending and breakage and the strain guage located proximally for determining the distraction force. Many prototype distractors have been used in developing this method. Also since there may be other models on the market the surgeon should carefully follow the manufacturer's instructions in each instance. A wing nut may be used to prevent slippage of the distal pins.

The distraction technique for arthroscopic surgery is done in the following manner (Figure 6-4). An Acufex pin $3/16$ of an inch in diameter is placed into the tibia above, and another into the os calcis below, along the lateral aspect of the extremity. This size is recommended, since a more rigid pin of larger diameter may exert undue force on the ligamentous structures. The upper pin is placed about $1\frac{3}{4}$ inches to 2 inches above the ankle joint, and drilled just behind the anterior tibial crest away from the anterior tibial artery. The Acufex cannula may be desirable to protect the soft tissues. The fibula should not be used as it can fracture, or the pin may cut out. The pin can also slip behind the tibia, if the fibula is used, and do damage in that area. The lower pin is placed immediately adjacent to the peroneous longus tendon and into the os calcis, about $\frac{1}{2}$ inch anterior to its posterior border and about $\frac{1}{2}$ inch above the inferior border of this bone (Figure 6-5). This avoids cutting out, when distraction is applied. The pins are inserted until good purchase is obtained. They should not exit beyond the medial cortex. The pin position in

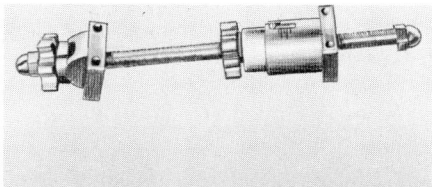

Figure 6-4. The distractor is shown. This model was designed to incorporate all the best features of previous models. A wrench is not necessary for efficient distraction. The strain gauge controls the proper tension, and the hinge at the distal end reduces pin bending and breakage (Acufex).

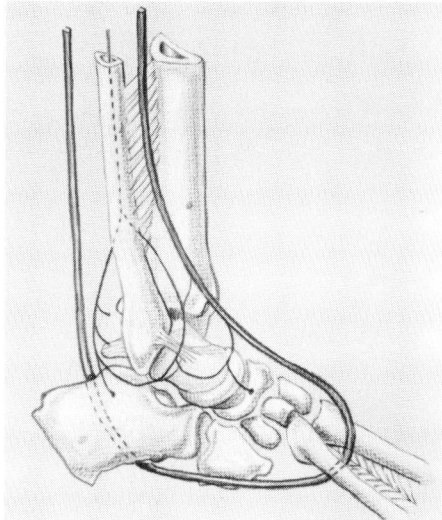

Figure 6-5. This diagram illustrates proper pin placement.

the os calcis can be determined by exploration with a hypodermic needle to outline the borders of that structure. Distraction is then applied slowly, up to about 4mm to 5mm. With the arthroscope then in place, more distraction is slowly and periodically applied during the procedure, until the joint is open to about 7mm to 8mm beyond normal. This should be about the maximum amount of distraction necessary. It appears that, as anesthesia time increases, there may be an elastic deformation of the ligaments, which allows more distraction than initially obtained. This should not continue beyond minimal bending of the pins or the proper force as shown by the distractor strain gauge. It is suggested that distraction not be maintained for more than approximately 45 to 60 minutes to avoid excessive and unnecessary stretching of the ligaments (35 to 50 pounds is recommended).

Distraction on the medial side can be used. The advantage is that the device is on the opposite side of that of the instruments when performing surgery. This was employed on occasion, early in the second series, but it was found that it was more comfortable for the surgeon with distraction applied on the lateral aspect of the joint. This is perhaps due to the anatomical configuration of the tibiotalar joint and the fact that the joint space opens with greater ease in the manner advocated. Through and through pins with double distraction (medial and lateral) may be employed occasionally in extremely tight ankle joints, as in cases of capsulitis, fibroarthrosis or degenerative arthritis. Also, placing the pin through the talus and tibia may be indicated in this situation.

Placement of the pins into the talus has been suggested routinely by some orthopedic surgeons. This has been avoided by the author because of the bulk of the malleoli on either side of the ankle joint, the neurovascular structures on the medial side, and also because of the danger of entering the subtalar joint and causing damage. The device would also be in the way of the instruments when triangulation in the tibiotalar articulation is performed, utilizing the anterolateral approach with other portals. Simultaneous exploration of the subtalar joint may be desired and is another reason for placement of the pin into the os calcis on the lateral side. An exception noted for pin placement into the talus would be for employing distraction and then compression, when doing an arthroscopic ankle arthrodesis. Also, as stated in cases of advanced capsulitis and fibroarthrosis, the talus may be chosen to more directly distract the ankle and avoid involvement of the subtalar joint when it is not necessary to do so. Should this pin placement be considered necessary it is important to select the proper site. According to Morgan (Chapter XII), "The distal pin is driven from medial to lateral into the body of the talus, beginning from a skin puncture placed just inferior and slightly anterior to the tip of the palpable medial malleous." X-rays are recommended to be sure that the pins have not violated the talocalcaneal joint.

Arthroscopic Technique

The ankle joint can be entered immediately as desired, or the distraction apparatus can be utilized at the beginning of the procedure, at the discretion of the surgeon. Injection of 0.5% Marcaine with epinephrine 1 to 200,000 is done at the portal sites to further reduce interarticular bleeding. A 16 gauge needle is placed into the joint. Repeated distention is suggested to stretch the capsule and gain more space. A small skin incision is then made, usually anterolaterally, with a drainage needle placed anteromedially. The distended joint capsule can be easily palpated for reference. With distraction, there is more room to enter the joint safely, without doing damage to the articular cartilage. A sharp obturater and cannula are then carefully placed into the joint. With the arthroscope in place, irrigation can be maintained by continuous infusion with a syringe monitored by the assistant. An overhead continuous inflow can be employed using a 1000cc bag of saline one meter above the level of the ankle. One cc of epinephrine 1 to 200,000 is instilled into the saline solution to further reduce intraarticular bleeding. Schonholtz[1] has recommended a simple blood pump for delivery of the saline, which is used at a pressure setting of 30mm of mercury to aid in managing inflow at arthroscopy. When this system is completed, initial viewing of the joint can be accomplished. The anatomical structures within the normal ankle joint were described in Chapter III. Further portal placement, wherever desired, is enhanced by placing a spinal needle in that area to gain optimum position and direction. After the desired inflow of fluid has been established, a probe is inserted into the joint on the opposite side for initial examination. In most cases, the shaver may be necessary to debride and eliminate chronic proliferative synovial tissue, which often obstructs the surgeon's view. There are a significant number of cases where an extensive synovectomy must be done. Then surgery is carried out, employing the appropriate portals and instruments.

Portals

In this author's experience, there are at least nine distinct portals of approach that should be considered (Figure 6-6). Each has its individual application for use in the various aspects of arthroscopic surgery of the ankle. Some are commonly or routinely used, and others are reserved for specific purposes when demand for them is required. Each will be discussed separately and the indications for the use of each will be illustrated. The need for a working knowledge of all approaches is obvious. There are three anterior portals: anterolateral, anteromedial, and anterocentral. An accessory portal can be used adjacent to the first two (i.e., an anterolateral accessory portal and an accessory anteromedial portal). These were also described by Schonholtz.[1] Accessory portals are no longer as necessary, in this author's opinion, as they were before the distraction method was developed. With distraction, the instruments (and arthroscope) can cross the joint with more ease from one side to the other side.

The posterolateral approach is immediately adjacent to the Achilles tendon and posterior to the peroneal tendons about a centimeter below the joint line. The posteromedial approach (also next to the heel cord) has been described by Chen[2] and used by him on only five occasions. Generally it is not recommended because of the obvious proximity of the posteromedial neurovascular bundle.

Employment of this approach, however, is possible, and may be required on rare occasions by an experienced arthroscopic surgeon, should triangulation in the posterior compartment be necessary. An example of this would be for the removal of a broken instrument fragment lodged in that area that could not be removed via the anterior portals. In some cases, when removal of loose bodies from this location is required in a tight ankle joint, where access from anterior cannot be obtained, an arthrotomy may be a wiser choice.

The transmalleolar portals are employed when adequate access to lesions of the talar dome for drilling or instrumentation cannot be adequately accomplished from the other portals. (Another transosseous approach for drilling was done on one occasion by the author through the anterior tibia when direct access to the lesion could not be obtained by the transmalleolar portals.)

The exact placement of each of the soft tissue portals is located with a hypodermic needle after the arthroscope is placed in its initial approach.

Anterolateral Approach

The anterolateral portal enters the joint between the fibula and talus about 0.5cm to 1cm distal to the joint line. It is adjacent and lateral to the common extensor tendon and extensor brevis (Figure 6-7). This is the classic or main diagnostic portal of the ankle joint, just as is the anterolateral (or inferolateral) portal of the knee, the main portal of that joint. The arthroscope is placed here, at least initially, and often the position is alternated between the arthroscope and instruments and with other portals as is neces-

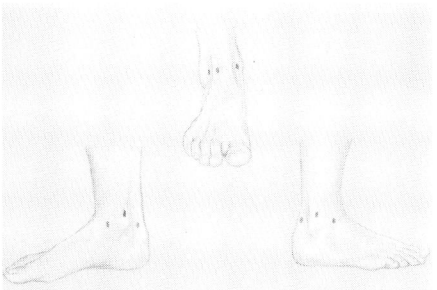

Figure 6-6. Portal placement as shown on the anterior, lateral, and medial views of the ankle. The posteromedial portal is seldom used except for rare indications by those skilled in ankle arthroscopy.

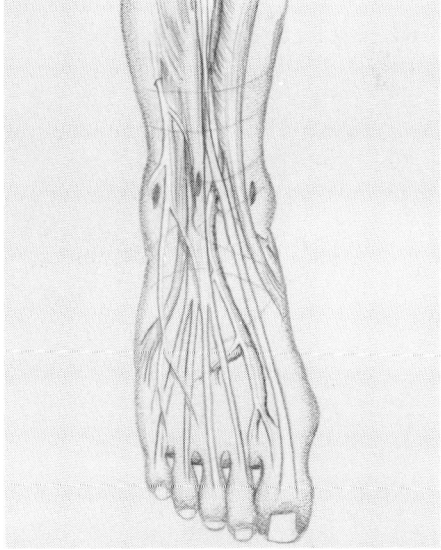

Figure 6-7. Portal placement in relation to superficial anatomic structures in the anterior ankle. (Modified from Drez, Guhl and Gollahan.)

sary. An adjacent accessory portal distal to the anterolateral portal can be determined by a spinal needle or hypodermic needle, if one has to triangulate on the lateral side of the joint between the fibula and talus. A distance of about 2cm should be maintained between these portals of entry. Also, damage to the superficial neurovascular structures (superficial peroneal nerve) should be avoided by marking them on the skin prior to surgery. The same technique is required in the accessory approach when performed on the medial side of the joint.

Anterocentral Approach

The anterocentral portal was described by Drez, Guhl, and Gollehon in 1981.[3,4,5] This portal was considered unnecessary and even dangerous by some at that time. However, when distraction is employed, there is a distinct advantage with greater ease of passage of instruments or the arthroscope from the anterior to the posterior compartment. This is because of the different degrees of concave curvature of the dome of the talus in the medial-lateral or coronal plane. This is illustrated in the chapters on gross and arthroscopic anatomy. Passage of instruments (or arthroscope) from the anterior to the posterior compartment is usually more difficult from the other anterior approaches because they must transcend the small "hump" on either side of the talar dome (Figure 6-8).

Triangulation from the anterior ankle to the mid-or posterior compartment is better therefore with the arthroscope inserted anterolaterally (anteromedially) and the instruments inserted through the anterocentral approach. This is particularly true in a relatively tight joint where limited distraction is available. In unstable joints, triangulation utilizing the anterolateral and anteromedial portals is a lesser problem. Also, if only a diagnostic arthroscopy of the ankle joint is desired, and especially if done under local anesthesia, a small diameter arthroscope (2mm to 3mm) may be used through the anterocentral approach. An adequate examination may then be performed without distraction, in a relatively loose joint. On occasion, a 70 degree oblique arthroscope can be passed through the anterocentral approach for viewing the entire posterior compartment. The anteromedial portal (as compared to the anterolateral approach) is another alternative for ease of passage to the posterior compartment because of the notch in the anterior tibial lip adjacent to the medial malleolus (See Chapter III).

The anterocentral approach (slightly lateral) has been best accomplished in the author's experience in the following way. A small vertical incision of 4mm to 5mm in length is made directly over the common extensor tendon at the level of the joint line (See Figure 6-7). The skin and subcutaneous tissue is spread with a small curved cryle instrument or hemostat and the extensor tendon is then pushed medially, "dragging" the other structures over about 1.0cm to 1.5cm in the medial direction. The neurovascular bundle is pushed well away towards the medial side of the joint, ahead of the extensors. The joint is then entered from a central position. A plastic cannula may be used to hold this placement and protect the vital structures. This appears to be easier and less dangerous than going between the extensor hallucis plus the ante-

Portals and Techniques 57

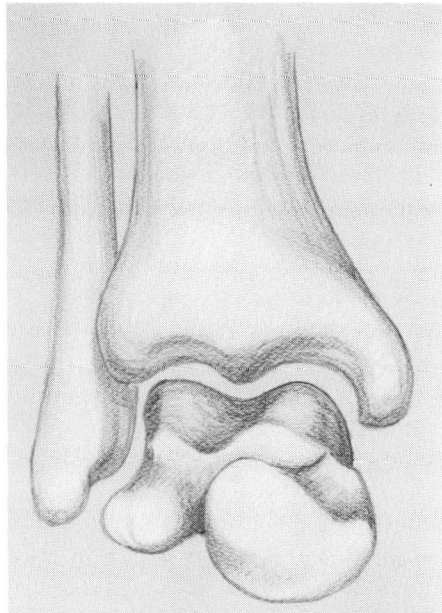

Figure 6-8. An ankle diagram of an early mammalian form demonstrating an exaggerated example of the ridges and the groove in the mid portion of the talus, in the anterior-posterior or sagittal plane. This configuration is present to a varying lesser degree in the human ankle, accounting for the greater ease of the anterocentral approach in many ankles. (Modified from Kelikian.)

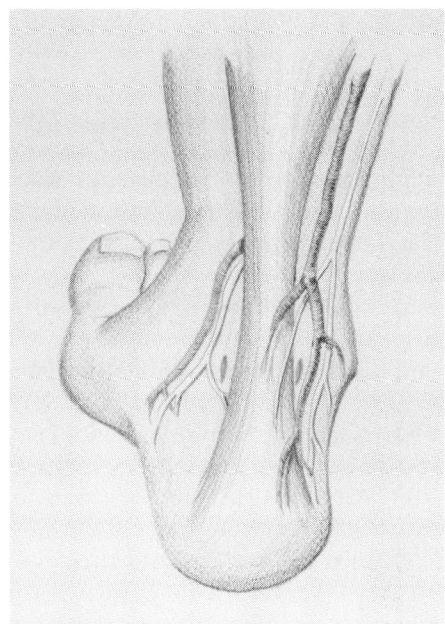

Figure 6-9. Portal placement in the posterior ankle, in relation to superficial anatomic structures. (Modified from Drez, Guhl, and Gollahan.)

rior tibial tendon, thus pushing laterally the big extensors with the nerve and artery. In the majority of cases, after distraction was employed, this approach was used and no problem was encountered when following the procedure in the above described manner. However, the surgeon must always keep in mind the proximity of the dorsal pedal artery and the anterior tibial nerve. Care must be taken not to stray further toward the center of the ankle.

Anteromedial Portal

The anteromedial portal enters the ankle between the medial malleolus and talar dome 0.5cm to 1cm distal to the joint line, just medial to the extensor hallucis longus and anterior tibial tendon (See Figure 6-7). The notch of the medial tibial plafond (Chapter III) may allow easier passage of the arthroscope or instruments to the posterior compartment. An adjacent accessory medial approach can be employed in the same manner, as when operating on the opposite side. When using the accessory approaches, care must be taken to place the portals far enough apart. Repeated entry here, especially with motorized equipment, should be avoided. There is minimal soft tissue between the skin and capsule in the area of the anterior portals, and sinuses can easily form and lead to infection.

Posterolateral Approach

The posterolateral approach is adjacent to the Achilles tendon and behind the peroneal tendons, slightly below the level of the joint line (Figure 6-9). The level of entry in the joint is determined externally by location — 0.5cm above the tip of the medial malleolus and 1cm above the tip of the lateral malleolus. Entry for these approaches can also be determined, when viewing from the anterior compartment, by placing a small spinal needle adjacent and lateral to the achilles tendon and at the level suggested above. The joint must be adequately distracted and distended.

This technique was not easily performed before the distraction method and ankle holder were employed. The standard method of triangulating to gain access to the posterior compartment is with the arthroscope anterolateral and the operating instruments anterocentral or anteromedial. Viewing could be done through the posterolateral portal when required, and instrumentation carried out via the anterior approaches or visa versa. If multiple approaches or extensive instrumentation are employed, plastic cannulas are of value in protecting the skin and soft tissues, thus lessening the chance for the development of a sinus and subsequent infection. A bridge for the purpose of exchanging the position of the arthroscope and operating instruments from one portal to another, as done in the shoulder, is suggested. When utilizing the posterolateral approach, one should avoid entering the subtalar joint (Figure 6-10) or causing damage to the sural cutaneous nerve and the short saphenous vein.

Trans-Achilles Tendon Approach

Recently Ewing and Ferkel[6] described the use of the trans-achilles tendon approach. The author has no experience with this to date, but it deserves consideration for the "complete" arthroscopic examination and arthroscopic surgery of the ankle joint.

Transmalleolar Approaches

The transmalleolar portals are employed on occasion to give better access to certain lesions of the talar dome. It would be required on the medial side more often than the lateral. This is because the lateral talar dome lesions are located more anterior than those on the medial side, and because the lateral malleolus is further posterior than the medial malleolus. This should be considered when utilizing the operating instruments, such as the drill, burr, or curette, to obtain an angle that is as close as possible to being perpendicular to the lesion (as described below). One is therefore able to get at the base of a crater adequately without scuffing or damaging the adjacent or healthy articular cartilage. When selecting this approach, the initial Kirschner wires are inserted about 2cm to 3cm above the joint in a line that

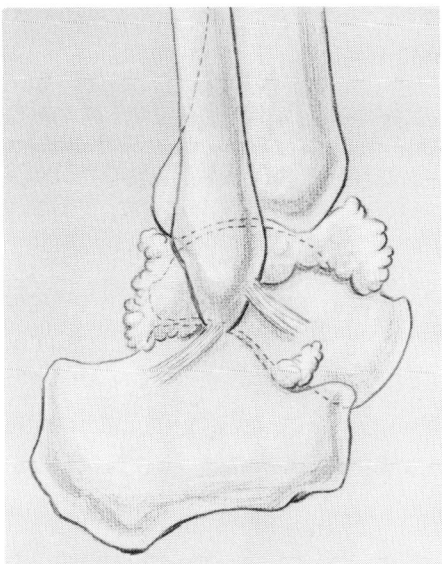

Figure 6-10. This diagram shows the extent of the anterior and posterior ankle joint recesses and the proximity of the subtalar joint and ankle joint when considering the posterolateral portal. (Modified from Kelikian.)

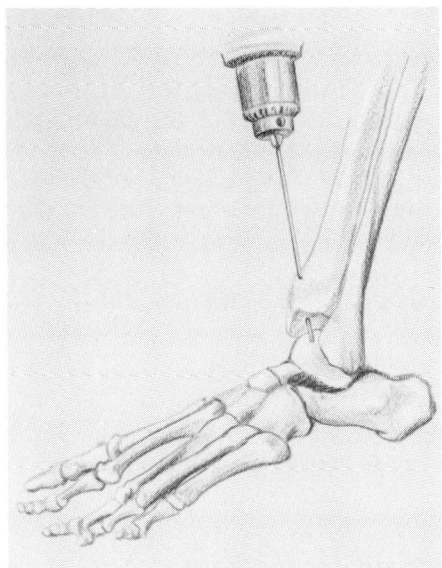

Figure 6-11. An illustration of the transmalleolar portal for drilling with an .062 Kirschner wire.

bisects the malleolus, as viewed from the medial or lateral side. They are then inserted in a distal direction and angled so they are perpendicular to the tangent of the lateral or medial curve of the dome of the talus where the lesion is located (Figure 6-11). Kirschner wires of .062 diameter may be used for drilling intact lesions of the talar dome under arthroscopic control, with the joint distracted. It is best to create a canal just slightly larger than the K-wires so that they can slip in or out of these holes with ease and reduce the risk of breakage.

The technique that was originally used by the author can be very difficult, and the wires often do not exit from the malleoli where desired or anticipated. Therefore, the use of the arthroscopic anterior cruciate ligament guide is important for accurate placement when employing this technique (Figure 6-12). Multiple drill holes can be made by placing two wires adjacent to each other in the medial-lateral plane, and then flexing and extending the talus in each direction (Figure 6-13). The wires are placed through slightly larger holes (more than 0.62), as indicated above. In this manner, a double row of holes, that is, from 4 to 10, can be made in the lesion of the talus. This is illustrated in Chapter X.

Another variation employing the transmalleolar approach may be considered. In this variation, a .062 Kirschner wire is placed accurately with the anterior cruciate ligament guide under arthroscopic control, while the joint is distracted. The exact desired exit can be obtained through the malleoli. A 5mm cannulated reamer (no larger) can then be advanced from a proximal

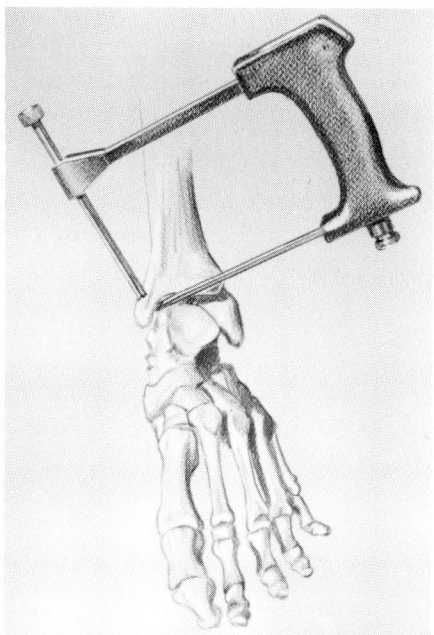 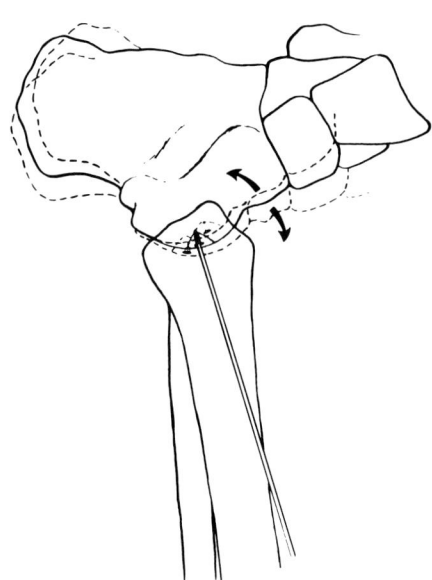

Figure 6-12. An illustration of the use of the arthroscopic anterior cruciate ligament guide for accuracy in portal placement and instrumentation of the defects of the talar dome.

Figure 6-13. This shows placement of multiple drill holes utilizing transmalleolar approaches.

position over the wire, creating a canal where desired. Another technique is to employ graduated drills, increasing in size to 5 mm. Care must be exercised in placement to avoid a potential fracture of the malleolus. Small operating instruments can then be passed down the canal for curetting, drilling, and abrading lesions of the talus. The difficulty and potential cartilage damage or scuffing from inadequate use of the anterior or posterior portals can be avoided. The edge of this canal should be chamfered or radiolysed by a power driven burr to eliminate sharp edges.

The techniques demonstrated above should be followed carefully in detail, especially regarding pin size, placement, and portal development as illustrated. The ankle holder used in conjunction with the bean bag has been designed for optimal ankle positioning. Allowance has been made for individual consideration of variation in body build. Placement of the extremity should be done with regard for the neurovascular status.

Alternate Techniques

There are two alternate techniques the surgeon may choose, should distraction not be desired. When contemplating choices, all that was discussed previously in this text regarding the superficial structures, gross and arthroscopic anatomy of the ankle joint, and the portals of approach should be kept in mind.

The first method has been shown by Andrews[7] (Figure 6-14). The extremity is placed in a knee holder and the end of the operating table is dropped 90 degrees, with the leg and ankle hanging over the side. This allows some distraction by gravity but not as much "controlled" separation of the joint as described in the mechanical distraction method. The foot and ankle can then be placed in the operating surgeon's lap and protected with drapes. There is some increased difficulty triangulating around the entire joint and especially utilizing the posterior approaches. Andrews recommended placing the inflow needle posterolateral, in cases when removing loose bodies by pushing them forward with a spinal needle inserted posteriorly.

Another alternate technique is presented as it has been decribed by Parisien.[8] It was designed initially for treatment of osteochondritis dissecans and osteochondral fractures. This technique does not require the distractor and ankle holder, but one must have the proper recommended instruments. (See Chapter V) There are advantages and also limitations. One should choose the technique fitting the particular circumstance.

The lateral decubitus position is used with the body tilted slightly posterior (Figure 6-15). The ankle to be operated on is elevated on a well padded box, as illustrated. With the ipsilateral hip rotated externally, the anterior aspect of the ankle is exposed for placement of the three approaches. The posterolateral portal is done with the hip in internal rotation. A disposible cannula with a side port inflow, placed through one of the two anterior approaches, has made the use of a drainage needle through a third anterior portal unnecessary. Complete evaluation is done by alternating the arthro-

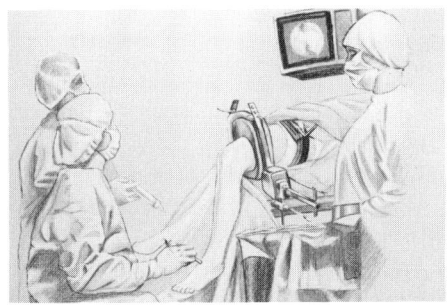

Figure 6-14. This shows the position of a patient on the operating room table for the first alternate technique (Andrews).

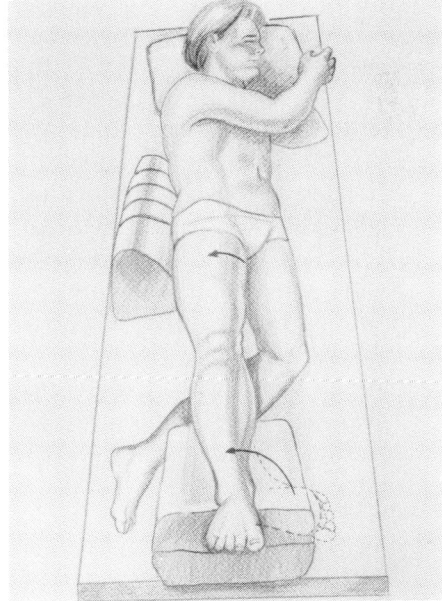

Figure 6-15. This shows the position of a patient on operating table for the second alternate technique. (Modified from Parisien.)

scope and spinal needle (for probing and irrigation), between the anteromedial and anterolateral portals.

Instrumentation is done through a disposible cannula with the ankle and foot in marked plantar flexion. When a lesion is encountered in the articular cartilage, it is scooped out with a banana knife. By excising the most anterior part of the lesion, the posterior portion is more accessible to surgical instrumentation. Curretage and abrasion is then carried out with small instruments. The technique must be performed with care and accuracy. The extremity is then placed in internal rotation as shown for ease of viewing the posterior compartment through a posterolateral portal.

Summary

In summary with the employment of these new techniques, there is more space to work efficiently in the ankle joint for diagnostic and treatment purposes. Alternate methods for performing ankle arthroscopy have been illustrated. The distinction method may be choosen by the orthopedic surgeon who poses an adequate experience and background in arthroscopic srugery and when the indications are clearly understood. Many advantages are described which should yield the best ultimate results. This method has been done safely by the author and no direct major complications have been encountered in 58 cases in this series and a total of 99 cases at the time of this publication.

References

1. Schonholtz GJ: Arthroscopic Surgery of the Shoulder, Elbow, and Ankle. Springfield. Charles C. Thomas, 1986.
2. Chen Y. Arthroscopy of the ankle joint. In: Arthroscopy of Small Joints. New York. IGAJU-SHOIN, 1985.
3. Drez D, Guhl JF, Gollahan DL: Ankle Arthroscopy: Technique and Indications. J Foot & Ankle 2:138-142, 1981.
4. Drez D, Guhl JF, Gollahan DL: Ankle Arthroscopy: Techniques and Indications. Clin in Sports Med 1(1):35-45, 1982.
5. Gollahan DL, Drez D: Arthroscopic Surgery Update, McGinity J. ed. 14 (15): 161-173 Text: Aspen Systems Corp 1985.
6. Ewing and Ferkel: Personal communication, 1987.
7. Andrews JR: Seminar — The American Foot and Ankle Society, January 1987, San Francisco, CA.
8. Parisien JS: Arthroscopic Treatment of Osteochondral Lesions of the Talus. Am J Sports Med 14(3):211-217, 1986.

CHAPTER 7

INDICATIONS AND CONTRAINDICATIONS

George J. Schonholtz, M.D.

During the past half decade, arthroscopic surgery of the ankle has become increasingly more useful, and the indications for its employment have widened to a considerable degree. At the time of this writing, indications and contraindications continue to be developed and revised as more procedures are being successfully accomplished. Refinement of techniques also continues.

Before undertaking any arthroscopic procedure of the ankle, a full, clinical evaluation is a necessity. This includes a complete history and physical examination, the x-ray studies outlined in Chapter IV, and laboratory tests, as indicated.

A preliminary trial of conservative care is always a sound practice, depending on the specific situation. Cast immobilization, an ankle support, anti-inflammatory medications, physical therapy, and an occasional injection of steroid medication should always be considered prior to arthroscopic surgery. With conservative treatment, many ankles will become asymptomatic and not require further treatment.

Indications

Perhaps the primary indication for arthroscopic surgery of the ankle joint is the lack of a specific diagnosis following a complete workup. This is especially true when associated with absence or poor response to conservative measures. Often, a chondral fracture or soft tissue pathology, previously unsuspected, is discovered. The more specific indications are as follows:

Soft Tissue Pathology: (1) local synovitis; (2) soft tissue impingement syndromes; (3) "meniscoid" formation; (4) generalized synovitis (posttraumatic); (5) synovitis-infectious (pyarthrosis); (6) synovial chondromatosis; (7) pigmented villonodular synovitis; (8) rheumatoid synovitis; (9) fibroarthrosis; (10) capsulitis; (11) intraarticular adhesions.

Chondral and Osteochondral lesions: (1) Osteochondral talar dome fractures (osteochondritis dissecans); (2) other osteochondral fractures; (3) loose bodies; (4) chondral lesions (chondral fractures, chondral necrosis, chondromalacia); (5) osteophytes (anterior and posterior impingement syndromes).

Arthritic Conditions: (1) Degenerative; (2) Posttraumatic, following intraarticular or extraarticular fractures; (3) rheumatoid; (4) postinfectious.

Other Indications: (1) Instability, especially lateral; (2) joint destruction, requiring ankle fusion; (3) reflex sympathetic dystrophy; (4) foreign bodies.

Soft Tissue Pathology

Increased awareness of the role of synovitis, soft tissue impingement syndromes, and the "meniscoid" lesion as the cause of ankle symptoms has only recently come about, following arthroscopic evaluations. These lesions can usually be managed by standard arthroscopic methods. Distraction techniques are at times useful in tighter ankles and where access is difficult.

Generalized, posttraumatic synovitis, synovial chondromatosis, pigmented villonodular synovitis, fibroarthrosis, and capsulitis and extensive adhesions are best managed arthroscopically. Utilization of the distraction method, as previously outlined in Chapter VI, is especially valuable to allow a more complete resection of pathological tissue and the utilization of larger instruments, such as large motorized shavers and basket forceps, which, in turn, expedite the procedure. In these entities, arthroscopic surgery is especially preferable to open methods, due to easier rehabilitation. Furthermore, any method of treatment may require a repeat synovectomy in perhaps 10% of cases. Due to the necessity, on occasion, for revisions, arthroscopic management is certainly more desirable.

As in other joints, chronic and acute infectious processes of the ankle may be managed arthroscopically. This is especially true when generalized, debilitating, medical conditions coexist. The standard methods of debridement, extensive lavage, and placement of egress and/or ingress catheters can be accomplished easily, utilizing arthroscopic techniques. A repeat procedure may be required if signs and symptoms do not recede within 48 hours of the initial surgery, especially when dealing with acute pyarthrosis. Distraction methods should not be employed here for fear of introducing the organisms into bone.

Chondral and Osteochondral Lesions

One of the most rewarding exercises in arthroscopic surgery of the ankle joint is the management of talar dome fractures (osteochondritis dissecans). Most of these lesions can be treated successfully utilizing arthroscopic techniques. This is preferable to open methods, especially when large, multiple incisions or osteotomy for exposure is required.

Lesions 1cm in diameter or less located anteriorly on the dome of the talus can be managed utilizing simple triangulation techniques. Larger lesions, located more posteriorly on the dome of the talus, may require distraction techniques. In an anterolateral lesion, a small arthrotomy incision may suffice, without significantly increasing rehabilitation time and morbidity.

Loose bodies of the ankle joint are easily removed arthroscopically. Depending on size, number, and position, distraction techniques may or may not be required. As is the case elsewhere, in spite of all efforts on the part of the surgeon, a repeat procedure may be necessary later to remove originally missed fragments or newly formed loose bodies.

The management of chondral lesions of the ankle is especially amenable to arthroscopy. In general, loose chondral material is debrided by the techniques described elsewhere in this text. Chondral lesions of the tibial plafond are best treated utilizing mechanical distraction techniques. Indeed, they may go undetected during the procedure unless the joint is distracted. Impinging osteophytes, especially those located anteriorly, can be effectively managed arthroscopically. This is true especially for the typical anterior impingement syndrome involving the lower tibia. Osteophytes located in the talar neck and elsewhere are probably best removed by a limited arthrotomy, particularly if they are large.

Arthritic Conditions

The various types of arthritis of the ankle joint, including degenerative, posttraumatic, rheumatoid, and postinfectious, have all been treated successfully utilizing arthroscopic techniques, albeit in small numbers at the time of this writing.

The actual findings are usually composed of several combinations of specific pathology. It is not unusual to discover synovitis, adhesions, loose bodies, areas of chondral necrosis or chondromalacia, osteophytes, as well as articular cartilage erosion down to bone in a single ankle. For this degree of involvement, it may be asking too much of arthroscopic surgery. Nevertheless, if each individual pathologic lesion is managed effectively in turn, some degree of improvement may be expected. Distraction techniques are especially helpful in this type of case.

With special reference to rheumatoid disease of the ankle joint, the main pathology may be cartilage necrosis of the talar dome, rather than synovitis. Synovitis may not be as evident as would be expected from extrapolating from the experience gained from arthroscopy of other joints. Rheumatoid arthritis may affect the subtalar joint, as well as the ankle joint, further clouding the clinical picture.

Other Indications

A method to stabilize the ankle, following disruption of the lateral ligaments, has been presented recently. Although technically possible, the final verdict must await longterm followup and comparison with more orthodox surgical techniques.

A few cases of ankle arthrodesis have been accomplished arthroscopically. This procedure, which is discussed elsewhere in the text, will most likely be indicated in the few patients who cannot be treated otherwise. These patients include those with poor skin, extensive scars, vascular, neurologic, or other complications, for whom open procedures would be more risky. In order to stand the test of time, however, the percentage of fusion must equal or be better than that accomplished by open means.

Arthroscopic surgery of the ankle joint may play a part in the management of reflex sympathetic dystrophy (RSD). Its primary value lies in the ability to rule out unsuspected pathology within the joint. Immediately following the procedure, an ipsilateral, sympathetic block is carried out. This is followed up with physical therapy and an oral medication regime, sometimes referred to as the "Triple Cocktail," which consists of a nonsteroidal, anti-inflammatory drug, Valium and Hydergine, 1mg, three times a day. Patience is required in managing these difficult problems. On rare occasions, a repeat sympathetic block and/or sympathectomy may be required. Distraction techniques, with additional pin placement, should be avoided when reflex sympathetic dystrophy is suspected.

Foreign bodies may be extracted from the ankle joint arthroscopically. The usual triangulation techniques used for osteochondral and chondral loose bodies are usually effective in removing them. A suction magnet device should be available when managing metallic, foreign, loose bodies. Iatrogenic loose bodies, secondary to instrument breakage, will be discussed further in Chapter XVI. Distraction techniques may be required, depending on the size and location of the foreign body.

Contraindications

Of course it may be argued that the only absolute contraindication to arthroscopic surgery of the ankle joint is ipsilateral below-knee amputation and arthrodesis. However, there are other contraindications — some absolute and others relative. Generalized infection elsewhere in the body, which does not involve the ankle, is an absolute contraindication to the procedure. Likewise, poor skin condition, including furuncles, recent lacerations, infection and rashes, are contraindications.

Partial ankylosis, severe fibrosis, and capsulitis are relative contraindications; however, with further development of distraction techniques, more of these patients will be candidates for arthroscopic surgery of the ankle joint.

Severe edema of the ankle may obscure landmarks and make the procedure very difficult. In addition, ankle edema may be secondary to generalized medical or vascular problems that require further investigation prior to surgery.

Before the operative procedure is undertaken, a careful neurologic and vascular examination should be carried out. Any neurologic or vascular defects should be documented and, if necessary, investigated prior to the procedure. Poor vascular status of the limb is usually a contraindication to the procedure.

Several advanced techniques, namely distraction and transmalleolar approaches, discussed in this text, may be contraindicated under certain circumstances. In children with open epiphyses, distraction and transmalleolar approaches are probably best avoided for obvious reasons. It has already been noted that these techniques are contraindicated when dealing with pyarthrosis, chronic infections, and, probably, reflex sympathetic dystrophy.

The distraction method may not be uniformly indicated. In the patient with a normally loose ankle, or where the pathology can be reached easily and manipulated with simple triangulation techniques, distraction should not be utilized, since the method adds still another layer of potential complications.

Discussion

In evaluating the indications for arthroscopic surgery of the ankle joint, one must try to assess the benefits of each individual procedure as it applies to specific pathology. Unfortunately, at the time of this writing no large series of cases is available for complete analysis. Nevertheless, some indications of effectiveness of therapy are emerging. It would appear that those procedures and techniques that have proven successful in the knee joint continue to prove successful in the ankle joint.

Within this author's experience the following pathological entities of the ankle joint have a good prognosis: (1) dome fractures of the talus (osteochondritis dissecans); (2) isolated chondral fractures; (3) loose bodies; (4) isolated "meniscoid" lesions, (5) anterior impingement spur; and (6) acute pyarthrosis.

The following lesions have a fair prognosis: (1) chondral necrosis; (2) chronic synovitis; (3) arthritis (all types); (4) posttraumatic adhesions; (5) reflex sympathetic dystrophy; (6) pathology involving previous, multiple open operations; and (7) severe, old ligament damage.

In the future, with refinement of our present techniques and the addition of new ones, it is hoped that many of the pathological entities in the latter list will be added to the former.

CHAPTER 8

DIFFERENTIAL DIAGNOSIS OF ANKLE PROBLEMS

William G. Hamilton, M.D.

Introduction

The chronically swollen, painful ankle can present a diagnostic challenge for any orthopedist. A thorough history, physical exam, and appropriate laboratory tests are an essential first step toward a sound diagnosis. Beyond these, a systematic approach to the problem may help simplify the maze that is often encountered with this patient.

It is useful to classify ankle problems as systemic, functional, periarticular or intraarticular. In other words, the classification depends upon whether the problem is due to systemic disease, the joint being used in a way that makes it painful, or a problem in the tissues around the joint or within the joint itself.

A bone scan is useful in determining whether the problem is osseous or soft tissue; and, if osseous, may localize the problem anatomically and suggest its nature, (stress fracture, osteoid osteoma, or degenerative joint disease).

A detailed list of possible causes for ankle pain is found in Table 8-1. Below some of the more common conditions encountered in every day situations are discussed.

Systemic

Many systemic diseases are associated with swelling and pain in the ankle. Among these diseases are:
  -Cellulitis.

-Charcot's joint; tabetic or syringomyelic.
-Circulatory, (claudication).
-Congestive heart failure.
-Diabetic arthropathy; neuropathic and infective.
-Gout (talagra) and pseudogout.
-Neurologic: lumbar disk disease; spinal stenosis or tumor; diastometamyelia; syringomyelia; amyotrophic lateral sclerosis; CMT disease; multiple sclerosis; muscular dystrophy.
-Osteoarthritis.
-Renal failure.
-Rheumatic diseases.
-Septic joint (especially gonococcus).
-Venous stasis. The left ankle will normally tend to swell more than the right because the left femoral vein passes under the aortic bifurcation to get to the vena cava, whereas the venous return in the right femoral vein is unobstructed.

Functional

The ankle, situated between the knee above and the foot below, is affected mechanically by abnormalities in either of these two joints:
-Anterior impingement will occur in the cavus foot of the dancer or athlete.
-Genu varum pronates the foot and genu valgum supinates it (in relation to the ankle).
-An incompetent, shortened, hypermobile first ray can pronate the foot, causing lateral impingement on the distal fibula.
-Leg length inequalities, if significant (greater than ½ inch), may contribute to ankle symptoms.
-Loss of subtalar motion, either congenital, degenerative, or post-traumatic, will place abnormal stresses on the tibiotalar joint.
-Posterior impingement often accompanies a pes planus.
-Pronation is common in runners.
-Rotatory abnormalities in the tibia (external tibial torsion will supinate the foot and internal torsion will produce pronation).

Periarticular

Anterior
-The anterior impingement syndrome (tibiotalar). Osteophytes may form on the anterior lip of the tibia, on the neck of the talus, or on both. The osteophytes may also break off and become loose bodies, either anchored by soft tissues or free in the joint.
-The anterior impingement syndrome involving only the the anterior rim of the medial malleolus against the medial shoulder of the talus. These anterior impingement osteophytes may lie in the capsular attachments to the neck of the talus, or even be extracapsular and thus hard to see with the arthroscope. It is helpful to take down the capsular insertion with a small

periosteal elevator or knife to be certain that you haven't missed one of these "hidden spurs." If there is any doubt, an x-ray taken at the end of the procedure will confirm an adequate cleanout.

-An occult osteoid osteoma in the tarsal navicular or neck of the talus can mimic an anterior impingement syndrome.

-A stress fracture of the neck of the talus or the tarsal navicular.

-Avascular necrosis of the talus (idiopathic or posttraumatic).

-A tear or partial tear of the anterior tibiofibular ligament with herniation of the joint capsule.[1]

-Sprain of the tibiofibular syndesmosis with avulsion of a small fragment from the tibial insertion of the anterior tibiofibular ligament. The "fragment of Tillot."

-Tendinitis or partial rupture of the anterior tibial tendon.

Medial

-Tendinitis or partial rupture of the posterior tibial tendon.

-A sesamoid bone in the posterior tibial tendon.

-An accessory ossicle at tarsal navicular or tip of the medial malleolus.

-A stress fracture of the sustentaculum tali.

Posterior-Medial

-The tarsal tunnel syndrome. This may be associated with abnormalities and anatomic variations within the tarsal tunnel, such as reduplicated arteries and nerves, accessory tendons and muscles (the flexor hallucis accessorius), retinacular cysts, or subtalar ganglia.

-Tendinitis or partial rupture of the flexor hallucis longus. "Dancer's Tendinitis." If severe, triggering of the great toe may be present (hallux saltans).

-A localized, fibrous, talo-calcaneal coalition is sometimes seen in this location.

-The posterior impingement syndrome of the ankle almost always occurs laterally. On rare occasions a large posterior-medial lip may be present on the back of the talus causing a posterior-medial impingement.

Posterior-Lateral

-Subluxation of the peroneal tendons, either partial or complete.

-Tendinitis or stenosis of the peroneal tendons.

-The posterior impingement syndrome involving (1) the os trigonum; (2) a trigonal process (Sticda's process); (3) a "marsupial meniscus"[2] (The marsupial meniscus is a true meniscus lying in the posterior-lateral ankle joint attatched to the tibial slip of the posterior talo-fibular ligament. It is a constant structure in marsupials and has been found occasionally in placentals, i.e., humans); or (4) a fracture or stress fracture of the trigonal process or of the os trigonum itself.

Lateral

-Residual ankle instability following sprain of lateral ligaments (positive "drawer sign" and talar tilt).

-Entrapment of capsule or ligament stump inside the lateral malleolus following sprain.

-Herniation of the capsule through a rent in the anterior talo-fibular ligament following sprain.

-The meniscoid of the lateral ankle (the "plica" of the ankle).[3]

-Tendinitis of the peroneus longus as it passes around the cuboid (may be associated with a sesamoid bone in the tendon).

-Subluxation of the cuboid.[4]

-Stress fracture, unicameral cyst, or osteoid osteoma of the os calcis.

-Fracture of the "beak" of the os calcis at the origin of the extensor digitorum brevis in the sinus tarsi.

-Osteophyte formation and impingement in the "bottom" of the sinus tarsi.

-Arthritis, coalition, or fibrosis of the subtalar joint resulting in loss or absence of normal subtalar motion.

-An accessory ossicle at the tip of the fibula or an avulsed fragment from a prior ankle sprain.

Idiopathic

-incisional neuromas from prior surgical procedures are often found on the anterior ankle and midfoot.

Intraarticular

-Congenitally flat talus, with or without tarsal coalition. The natural shape of the talus can range from quite circular to quite flat. The flat talus will naturally have a greatly decreased range of motion and will tend to impinge in plantar and dorsiflexion.

-Osteochondritis dissecans may be medial or lateral, posttraumatic or idiopathic, symptomatic if loose, but asymptomatic if intact. It is not uncommon to see old osteochondritis dissecans lesions that have healed spontaneously. An arthrogram will usually determine whether the fragment has loosened. If the dye on the x-ray enters the cavity, the hyaline cartilage overlying the lesion must be broken and the fragment loose.

-Loose bodies: These may be hard to identify, even with an arthrogram, because they tend to be small, often are cartilagenous, and may lie in the recesses of the ankle joint (they have been found in the flexor holluces longus tendon sheath tunnel).

-Articular damage: Early degenerative joint disease characterised by lost or damaged hyaline cartilage may follow trauma or repeated ankle sprains with loose ligaments and rotatory instability of the talus. In the early phases, this condition can be subtle, as symptoms may be present before cartilage space narrowing is seen on x-rays. A bone scan at this stage will usually give a characteristic appearance. A diffuse increased uptake outlining the joint is seen instead of the focused pattern usually found with discrete lesions.

Conclusion

If uncertain of the diagnosis, a bone scan is quite useful. It will determine whether the problem is osseous or soft tissue. If the scan is normal, it is helpful to try a series of 1cc injections of local anesthetic into various anatomical locations to determine the exact source of the pain. Once the site of the problem is known and a temporary response is obtained from the local anesthetic, an injection of corticosteroid can be tried if the problem is not intraarticular. If the bone scan was positive but the regular x-rays are normal, CAT and MR scans will often reveal pathology that cannot be seen on regular films.

References
1. Laughlin HL: Trauma. Philadelphia: W.B.Saunders, 1960, p. 341.
2. Hamilton WG, Sheskier S: The Marsupial Meniscus as a Cause of Posterior Impingement in Dancers. In preparation for Foot & Ankle.
3. Wolin I, Glassman F, Sideman S, Leventhal Z: Internal Derangement of the Talo-Fibular Joint of the Ankle. Surg Gyn & Ob 91:193, 1950.
4. Newell SG: The Cuboid Syndrome. The Physician and Sportsmedicine 9(4):71, 1981.
5. French's Index of Differential Diagnosis. PSB Publishing Co., Littleton, MA.
6. The Merck Manual, Merck and Co., Inc., Rahway, NJ, 14th Edition, 1982.

**Table 8-1.
Diseases Causing Ankle Pain**

There are a multitude of diseases, both common and rare, that can cause ankle pain.[5,6]

Polyarthritis of Unknown Etiology
    Adult-onset Still's disease
    Ankylosing spondylitis
*   Juvenile rheumatoid arthritis
    Palindromic rheumatism
    Reiter's syndrome
*   Rheumatoid arthritis

Connective Tissue Disorders
    Amyloidosis
    Eosinophilic fasciitis
    Polymyositis and dermatomyositis
    Scleroderma
    Systemic lupus erythematosis
    Vasculitis and necrotizing arteritis
        Cogan's syndrome
        Giant cell arteritis (including polymyalgia rheumatica)
        Goodpasture's disease
        Henoch schonlein purpura
        Hypersensitivity angiitis
        Polyarteritis nodosa
        Takayasu's (pulseless) disease
        Wegener's granulomatosis

Degenerative Joint Disease
    Primary (common in older athletes and dancers)
    Secondary (posttraumatic)
*   Ankle fractures
*   Avascular necrosis (AVN) of the talus following dislocation. (AVN of 27x29.1the talus can be symptomatic before it shows on normal x-rays.)

Disorders Frequently Associated With Arthritis
    Acromegaly
    Acute rheumatic fever
    Familial Mediterranean fever
    Haemophylia and allied disorders
    Intestinal bypass surgery
*   Psoriasis
    Regional enteritis
    Relapsing polychondritis
    Sarcoidosis
    Sickle cell disease
    Sjogren's syndrome
    Ulcerative colitis
    Whipple's disease
    Yersina enterocolitica infection

*Commonly occurring in the ankle region

Table 8-1. (cont.)

Known Infectious Agents
    Bacterial
        Anthrax
        Brucella
        Diptheria
        Erysipelas
*   Gonococcus (commonly affects the ankle)
        Haverhilia
        Kala-azar
        Leprosy
*   Lyme disease (treponema spread by the tick *Ixodes dammini*)
*   Meningococcus
        Mycoplasma pneumonia (Eaton's agent)
        Mycobacterium tuberculosis
*   Pneumococcus
        Pseudomonas pseudomallei
        Rat bite fever
        Salmonella
        Staphylococcus
        Streptobacillus monoliformis (Haverhill fever)
        Streptococcus
        Subacute and acute bacterial endocarditis
        Treponema pallidum (secondary syphilis)
        Treponema pertenue (yaws)
        Typhoid and paratyphoid fever
        Weil's disease (Leptospirosis)
    Rickettsial
    Viral
        Behcet's disease
        Chikungunya
        Echo virus infection
        Epidemic Australian arthritis
        Glandular fever (infectious mononucleosis)
        Infective and serum hepatitis
        Influenza
        Lymphogranuloma venerans
        Measles
        Mumps
        Poliomyelitis
        Psittacosis
        Rubella
        Smallpox

*Commonly occurring in the ankle region

Table 8-1. (cont.)

Known Infectious Agents (cont.)

    Fungal
      Actinomycosis
      Aspergillosis
      Blastomycosis
      Coccidioidomycosis
      Cryptococcosis (torulosis)
      Histoplasmosis
      Madeira foot (mycetoma pedis)
      Sporotricosis
    Parasitic and protozoan
      Amoebiasis
      Chylous arthritis
      Dracunculosis (Guinea-worm disease)
      Filariasis
      Trichiniasis

Neurogenic
*   Diastometamyelia
*   Neuropathic arthropathies (Charcot's Joints)
*   Congenital insensitivity to pain (familial dysautonomia)
*   Diabetes mellitus
*   Myelomeningococele
*   Syphilis
      Syringomyelia
*   Spinal cord tumors
*   Spinal disk disease
*   Spinal stenosis

Arthritis Associated with Known Biochemical or Endocrine Abnormalities
    Acromegaly
    Agammaglobulinemia
    Alcaptonuria (ocronosis)
    Apatite crystal disease
*   Chrondrocalcinosis (pseudogout)
    Fabrey's disease (glyco lipid lipidosis)
    Gaucher's disease
*   Gout
    Hemochromatosis
    Hyperlipoproteinemia (xanthoma tuberosum)
    Hyperparathyroidism
    Osteomalacia
    Rickets
    Scurvy (hypovitaminosis C)
    Thyroid acropachy
    Wilson's disease

*Commonly occurring in the ankle region

Table 8-1. (cont.)

Neoplasms
    Benign
*   Bone cyst (often found in the os calcis)
        Chondroblastoma
        Chondromyxofibroma
        Enchondroma
        Giant cell tumor
*   Nonossifying fibroma
*   Osteoblastoma
*   Osteochondroma
*   Osteoid osteoma
        Pigmented villonodular synovitis
    Primary malignant tumors
        Ewing's sarcoma
        Fibrosarcoma
        Chondrosarcoma
        Malignant fibrous histeocytoma
        Malignant giant cell tumor
        Malignant lymphoma of bone
        Mesenchymal chondrosarcoma
        Multiple myeloma
        Osteogenic sarcoma
        Synovioma
    Leukemia
    Metastatic malignant tumors (rare below the knee)

Allergy and Drug Reactions
    Drug induced lupus-like syndromes
        Hydralazine
        Procaine amide
    Hypersensitivity angitis
    Serum sickness

Inherited and Congenital Disorders
    Achondroplasia
    Angiokeratoma corporis difussum (Fabrey's disease)
    Arthrogryposis multiplex congenita
    Arthroonychodysplasia
    Arthroopthalmopathy
    Camptodactly
    Congenital insensitivity to pain
    Congenital talipes equinovarus
    Congenital vertical talus
    Cutis laxa
    Dysplasia epiphysalis multiplex
    Ehlers-Danlos syndrome
    Familial dysautonomia (Reiley-Day syndrome)
    Hurler's syndrome (gargoylism)
    Homocystinuria

*Commonly occurring in the ankle region

Table 8-1. (cont.)

Inherited and Congenital Disorders (cont.)

    Marfan's and other hypermobility syndromes
    Morquio-Brailsford osteochondrodystrophy
    Mucopolysaccaridoses
    Myositis ossificans progressiva
    Osteogenesis imperfecta
    Pseudoxanthoma elasticum
    Tumoral calcinosis
    Werner's syndrome

Miscellaneous Disorders

    Amyloidosis
    Biliary and alcoholic cirrhosis
* Avascular necrosis of bone
* Congestive heart failure
* Dependent edema (The left ankle will normally tend to swell more than the right because the left femoral vein passes under the aortic bifurcation to join the vena cava, whereas the venous return in the right femoral vein is unopposed).
    Disseminated lipogranulomatosis (Farber's disease)
    Erythema multiforme (Steven-Johnson's syndrome)
    Erythema nodosum
    Familial lipochrome pigmentary arthritis
    Hypertropic pulmonary osteoarthropathy
    Intermittent hydrarthrosis
* Juvenile osteochondritis
* Kohler's disease
    Multicentric reticulohisteocytosis
* Osteochondritis dissecans
* Osteoporosis
    Pancreatitis or pancreatic carcinoma
    Polymyalgia rheumatica
    Pigmented villonodular synovitis and tendinitis
    Relapsing panniculitis (Wever-Christian disease)
    Renal failure
    Sjogren's syndrome
    Steroid crystal-induced synovitis
    Subacute bacterial endocarditis
* Tarsal tunnel syndrome
* Tendinitis, fasciitis, bursitis, tenosynovitis
    Thrombotic thrombocytopenic purpura
* Venous stasis
    Synovial chondromatosis or osteochondromatosis

*Commonly occurring in the ankle region

CHAPTER 9

SOFT TISSUE (SYNOVIAL) PATHOLOGY

James F. Guhl, M.D.

Introduction

These lesions are synovial in origin in all but a few instances where capsular or ligament tissue may be involved. This pathology accounts for about one-third of the lesions in the ankle joint. The specific kinds of synovitis are rheumatoid synovitis, chronic synovial chondromatosis, pigmented villonodular synovitis, and others. There is also a chronic, nonspecific synovitis, which may be general or local. This type is secondary in most cases to some degree of trauma. A number of these soft tissue entities also occur coincidentally with chondral pathology, and only on occasion with a certain amount of instability. The latter is often minimal and in most cases is not a problem. Until recently, with mechanical distraction, these local soft tissue lesions (and chondral defects) were most difficult or impossible to diagnose except by an exploratory arthrotomy. It is obvious that this was not practical and a significant number of pathological entities could therefore not be appreciated or treated.

The types of synovial or soft tissue pathology are classified below and will be discussed under these headings.

Classification

Soft Tissue Pathology (Synovitis), Specific
Rheumatoid arthritis (synovitis).
Chronic synovial chondromatosis.
Pigmented villonodular synovitis.

Local.
   General.
Others.

Soft Tissue Pathology (Synovitis), Nonspecific
Chronic synovitis, general.
   Adhesions.
Chronic synovitis, local.
   Local Subacute (Chronic) Synovitis
   Soft tissue impingement
      Lateral.
      Medial.
      Posterolateral.
         Synovial nodule.
         Ganglion (interarticular, peroneal tendon sheath).
      Posterior.
         Pathological transverse tibiofibular ligament (tibial slip).
         Pathological meniscus of the ankle.
         Pathological labrum.

Infectious Synovitis

Soft Tissue Pathology (Synovitis), Specific
Rheumatoid Arthritis
Rheumatoid synovitis has the same picture when demonstrated arthroscopically as that seen in any other joint. In most cases there is synovial hyperplasia with villi, papillary formation, and necrosis. According to Schonholtz,[1] areas of articular cartilage necrosis of the tibial plafond and talar dome may be a feature, if not the main manifestation, of this disease in the ankle joint (Figures 9-1 and 9-2). He states that often synovitis is minimal.

Upon arthroscopic study, thickening, irregularity and proliferation of the synovial lining are at times brought out. In early cases, this may precede the osteoporosis and joint line narrowing seen on standard films. With the arthrogram, associated cartilage loss and lymphatic filling are seen in rheumatoid arthritis and variations of this disease. Synovial involvement may also be established by surface coil MR imagery. The treatment is arthroscopic synovectomy and debridement performed in the same manner as in synovial chondromatosis and pigmented villonodular synovitis. Rheumatoid arthritis has also been known to occur in the subtalar joint, perhaps more so than in the ankle joint.

Chronic Synovial Chondromatosis
Chronic synovial chondromatosis treated arthroscopically has also responded satisfactorily. This disease entity occurs in three stages. Stage I is a synovial involvement only with chondral fragments in the synovial membrane, a form of chronic synovitis. Stage II is an active synovial disease or a synovitis with chondral involvement along with numerous and often hundreds of chondral loose bodies in the joint. There is usually no osteoid

involvement in the early form, in which case the x-ray and bone scan would be negative. The arthrogram, CT scan, and MR would most likely be positive. Later in the second stage, there is bone formation within the synovial tissue and detached loose osteochondral fragments. The fragments are then seen on routine x-ray and are representative of a chronic synovial osteochondromatosis. In Stage III the synovitis becomes inactive and "burned out." This leaves multiple osteochondral loose bodies. In addition to these findings on x-ray, local articular cartilage damage and early degenerative arthritis are later seen due to mechanical dysfunction. Arthroscopically, there is a chronic synovitis with chondral or osteochondral fragments within the synovium, loose bodies, and later degenerative arthritis. The histopathology consists of chronic synovitis with extensive involvement of chondral or osteoid tissue in several stages of development as shown by staining techniques.

In the author's experience, response in these cases has often been dramatic with arthroscopic surgery. A synovectomy must be done in Stage I and Stage II, with loose body removal in the latter, requiring mechanical distraction and possible use of the posterolateral portal. In Stage III, debridement of the chondromalacia or arthritis (as indicated) and loose body removal are necessary, without a need for a synovectomy. The known recurrence rate of open surgery or arthrotomy is about 5%. No extensive experience with arthroscopic surgery has been reported to date, but it is reasonable to expect that the recurrence rate should be about the same or less. The difference, of course, is reduced morbidity and rehabilitation time when arthroscopic surgery is employed. This fact would also tend to make repeat surgery more acceptable, should there be a recurrence.

Pigmented Villonodular Synovitis

Pigmented villonodular synovitis can occur in the ankle, although probably less often than synovial chondromatosis. This disease entity responds equally as well as it did in the knee and other joints with arthroscopic treatment. The recurrence rate is about the same as that of chronic synovial chondromatosis. Clinically, the picture is a chronic synovitis with generalized swelling, aching, and pain aggravated by activity. All x-ray techniques are negative, except perhaps the arthrogram and surface coil MR imagery, according to a recent study by Beltram,[2] et al. (early reports). The swollen synovial tissue is seen, and this entity is further brought out by the "paramagnetic activity of the hemosiderin cells". Arthroscopically, there is a synovitis with a more advanced papillary formation and more pigment (hemosiderin) than in chronic hemorrhagic synovitis. Histologically, there should be an advanced cellular response with a fibrous reaction and multiple giant cells, pigmentation, and papillary formation. Treatment via arthroscopic surgery requires a synovectomy, which could quite adequately be done with distraction and the multiple portal approach.

Others

Ikeuchi[3] and Chen[4] have described some cases of gouty arthritis and Crohn's disease in Watanabe's book, *Arthroscopy in Smaller Joints*[4]. Again, a complete arthroscopic debridement should be done.

Synovitis, Nonspecific

Chronic Synovitis, General

Chronic posttraumatic synovitis or chronic hemorrhagic synovitis usually follows a major traumatic incident or often repeated minor trauma. This has previously been seen in the elbow and knee joint by the author, and it is associated with multiple bleeds or the overuse syndrome. This was noted in an elbow of a "class" swimmer and the elbow of a laborer who operated a pneumatic drill. Complete relief was obtained by extensive arthroscopic debridement, a short period of rest, and then general mobilization to full activity. Chondral damage was not an associated problem in the small number of cases in these joints to date. The same picture was later experienced in the ankle joint by this author.

The symptoms in the ankle joint, as in the other joints, are usually chronic generalized aching pain with minimal swelling, and generalized tenderness. Adequate medical evaluation should be employed for differentiation, since such entities as pseudogout and others can occur, as we have seen in one case. This is further pointed out in Chapter VIII and its appendix on differential diagnosis. Routine and special x-ray techniques are negative, except for perhaps the arthrogram, which may show synovial proliferation and irregularity. It may also be reflected by MR imagery. Conservative treatment may include heat modalities, antiinflammatory medications, an injection, if necessary, and perhaps a period of immobilization. This is followed by a rehabilitation program. Should this regime fail, surgical intervention is then employed.

Arthroscopically, the offending tissue appears as a chronically inflamed synovitis, including some papillary formation. Occasionally, there is some scattered hemorrhagic material and minimal pigment deposition. Chronic cartilage damage is usually not associated, except in advanced cases. Microscopically, a subacute or chronic synovitis with a cellular inflammatory response is all that is seen. The author has experienced satisfactory results with arthroscopic synovectomy.

Adhesions

The next type of soft tissue pathology is adhesion formation, which occurs on occasion, following mild to moderate ankle sprains or undisplaced fractures such as that of the distal fibula or medial malleolus. It appears that the fractures or ligament disruptions requiring open or closed reduction, or surgical repair of the latter, are not followed by adhesions (or the soft tissue impingement) as often as the less severe injuries. With displaced fractures or ligament tears, the interarticular blood escapes into the surrounding soft tissue. Also, it is removed when an open reduction and internal fixation are performed. In sprains and undisplaced fractures, there often is a hemarthrosis that is not aspirated, it is ultimately and usually absorbed by the synovium. In some cases, however, there is further exudate and swelling. This is followed by an extensive cellular response, fibrous tissue reaction, hyalinization, and, ultimately, chronic synovitis, which subsequently leads to extensive adhesion formation.

The symptoms in the cases seen to date are often more dramatic than those seen from other soft tissue entities mentioned above. On occasion locking may be seen with marked pain and relief when unlocking occurs. A feeling of instability is another symptom that has been interpreted as a chronic ligament disruption. In one patient, repair or reconstruction was requested. There was, however, no significant instability on x-ray examination. A loud clicking often is described by the patient and has been experienced by this examiner. Mild generalized swelling is seen with various areas of local tenderness. Sometimes motion may be limited or painful, as demonstrated in the case discussed.

The arthroscopic diagnosis is dramatic and explains the symptoms. There is usually an underlying chronic synovitis. Multiple bands of adhesions, of various degrees, are seen stretching from one side of the ankle to the other in an oblique, horizontal, or vertical plane (Figure 9-3). These are seen more commonly in the anterior ankle joint where there is more room. They occur to a lesser degree in the posterior compartment. An adhesion may be seen in the lateral talomalleolar area as a form of synovial impingement, but it is rarely noted on the medial side. There is also little room in the talocrural articulation. The numerous locations of these adhesions account for the generalized swelling and the points of pain and tenderness. Another arthroscopic finding that has been seen with adhesions is a groove in the articular cartilage of the anterior dome of the talus, corresponding directly to the path of the adhesion. These and other associated chondral defects may be responsible for the feeling of instability, locking and clicking.

Arthroscopic removal of the adhesions is accomplished by the use of the basket forceps, rongeur, and motorized debriders. Arthroscopic synovectomy may be necessary. The tissue forming the adhesions is tough and elastic arthroscopically, and histologically is seen in a more advanced stage of organization than chronic synovitis alone. Arthroscopic excision must be complete, since recurrence has been seen. Treatment of chondral defects, as described separately in this text, is also important. Precautionary measures should be taken postexcision, such as the use of interarticular epinephrine (0.5% Marcaine with epinephrine 1 to 200,000), with perhaps a steroid instilled at the conclusion of the procedure to prevent further bleeding (and a recurrence). Elevation, ice packs, and pressure dressings for 24 to 48 hours are advised. Aspirations should be performed if necessary. This is later followed by a proper postoperative rehabilitation program. Active range of motion and strengthening exercises and the timing of weight bearing is dictated by the degree of involvement in each individual case. (See Chapter XV).

Local Synovitis

Chronic Local Synovitis

Local synovitis usually occurs in the lateral talomalleolar joint and, in most cases, responds to arthroscopic debridement, if conservative treatment fails. Arthroscopic findings are local subacute or chronic synovitis, minimal papillary formation (Figure 9-4) and, occasionally, a few fibrous adhesions.

Before arthroscopic treatment is employed, this author feels that various forms of conservative treatment should be tried. At least two to three months from the onset should elapse, with a significant disability resulting, before arthroscopic surgery is chosen. The usual initial immobolization of these minor injuries is three to four weeks in a cast, depending upon the degree of strain or ligament disruption or the extent of the undisplaced fracture. This should be followed by proper rehabilitation: ankle supports, physical therapy with heat modalities, exercise, and antiinflammatory medications. Later, if synovitis persists, a steroid injection during the chronic stage is reasonable. Prior to arthroscopic intervention, further special x-ray techniques, as appear indicated in each case, should be employed. Emphasis should be placed on the preoperative stress films.

Synovial Impingement Syndrome

In cases of the synovial impingement lesion, there is, as seen at arthroscopy, a band of tough elastic synovial tissue. This is well localized and adheres to the roof of the lateral aspect of the ankle. It arises from the synovial recess located above the lateral talomalleolar joint in the tibiofibular articulation. On the surface of this lesion there is often seen scattered hemosiderin or pigment formation (Figure 9-5 and 9-6). Occurrence is most frequent on the lateral side of the ankle, but occasionally it occurs on the medial side (or both sides). In the latter instance, there is no synovial recess to serve as the origin, but it is made up of synovial, capsular, and ligamentous tissue. The lack of this point of origin and the reduced incidence of sprains on the medial side probably account for its less frequent occurrence at this location.

The clinical picture is usually tenderness over the lateral malleolus and anterior to that area, with intermittent local swelling. Pain is aggravated by inversion or eversion of the ankle and foot, and, sometimes, by dorsiflexion and plantar flexion. Routine x-ray techniques are generally of no diagnostic value. Arthrograms may indicate areas of associated articular cartilage damage, whereas one would not expect to see findings indicative of synovial involvement since this is a local disease or pathological entity. Mendelbaum[10] has shown the MR to be of diagnostic value as a noninvasive procedure in its detection (Figure 9-7). Further study needs to be done to establish this and its practical application.

Adequate arthroscopic diagnosis and treatment is enhanced by the mechanical distraction method. Chondral defects should be carefully searched for when treating a synovial impingement lesion. Their occurrence would depend upon the force at injury and somewhat on the degree of laxity as seen on stress films. Instability, however, is usually minimal or nonexistent, and these ankles often are quite stable, as noted in this series and by other investigators (Ferkel).[9] The tibial plafond should be the object of exploration, as well as the talar dome. Adequate and careful search is enhanced by also employing the posterior portal when probing or viewing. Use of the posterolateral portal would be indicated if the distraction obtained is inadequate and there is limitation of access to the posterior recess anteriorly. Tangential viewing with an oblique arthroscope, light dimming, and the use of methylene blue dye are also helpful. With these methods and careful probing, the areas of diseased and damaged cartilage are found. The probe is used to lift the affected cartilage away from the underlying bone. Basket forceps and motorized equipment are used to debride the area. These chondral defects should be carefully reconstructed to healthy cartilage with a perpendicular margin. The base should be debrided, abraded, and carefully drilled (See Chapter XI). The utilization of the posterolateral portal and transmalleolar approaches should be employed as necessary.

The chronic synovial impingement lesion is removed by the basket forceps, rongeur, curettes, and by motorized equipment. All involved tissue is excised down to the underlying cartilage. The synovial recess should be adequately debrided of impingement tissue, and any capsular or ligamentous tissue located anterolaterally should be excised. This material is tougher and more elastic than seen in the usual type of subacute or chronic synovitis. Histologically, there is subsynovial blood vessel proliferation, papillary hyperplasia, and chronic inflammation. The articular cartilage may show degenerative change (Figures 9-8 through 9-11) (Ferkel[9]). As more experience has been gained with cases of the impingement lesion, a pattern seems to have developed.

Posterolateral Impingement

In addition to the subacute synovitis at one extreme and the tough fibrous scarred type of lesion (meniscoid) at the other, there are other impingement lesions in between that have been seen to occur in at least two forms in the lateral talomalleolar compartment. The soft tissue or synovial impingement lesion extends from anterior to the posterior aspect of the ankle joint (described above). A second type was well localized in the posterolateral corner of the ankle. This lesion was found on several occasions as a small synovial nodule or cyst. The symptoms were invariably significant pain and tenderness in that area. In one case, the patient obtained relief by standing with her foot in inversion. The symptoms were clearcut, distinct, and dramatically relieved by excision. These lesions were essentially undiagnosed and therefore not treatable until the distraction device was employed. Arthrograms, as reported in the few cases (in our series to date), did not show any cystic outpouching or abnormality. When encountering this lesion at arthroscopy with the use of the probe, it seemed to be rather small, about the size of a small grape. As probing continued, more material was pulled from the posterolateral corner of the joint and removed. This structure seems to extend adjacent to the area and around the peroneal tendons and is similar to a Baker's cyst in the knee joint or a ganglion that may be visible on arthrography or ganglionography. These could be considered as interarticular ganglions of the ankle joint or as synovial cysts. All patients treated arthroscopically for this type of pathological structure were markedly improved (Figures 9-12 through 9-14).

The Meniscoid

The meniscoid, according to historical accounts, is a structure similar to, but apparently more advanced histologically than the usual synovial impingement lesion. It persists as a large band or adhesion in the lateral talomalleolar joint. Schonholtz[8] described this structure as torn and fibrosed fibers of the capsule and ligaments, as well as chronic synovial tissue. Chen[4] referred to the lesion in Watanabe's text *Arthroscopy of Small Joints*. Ikeuchi[10] described it as a band of connective tissue extending from the anterior talofibular ligament to the posterior talofibular ligament and largely free in the lateral talofibular articulation. Wolin et al[16] cited cases in several athletes and reported results of his series (Figure 9-15).

The term meniscoid has been adopted, since, upon gross examination, the tissue appears similar to a meniscus of the knee joint. This entity should be distinguished from the meniscus in the posterior compartment of the ankle described by Hamilton[12] as a posterior impingement lesion (Chapter VIII), and later as referred to in this discussion. The latter structure is histologically a true meniscus.

The author has noted three cases of the meniscoid and found them to be as described by Wolin,[6] Chen,[4] Ikeuchi,[3] and Schonholtz.[1] They seem to be larger than the synovial impingement lesion, lying free in the joint, and are not adherent to the overlying "roof" (or synovial recess) of the lateral tibiofibular joint. These pathological structures appear firm and tougher in consistency and contain more hypertrophied fibrous connective tissue.

Because of our limited knowledge, the meniscoid is discussed as a separate entity and as a more advanced lesion than the synovial impingement. Further study and subsequent reports may further simplify this classification.

The following description is taken from Wolin's[6] original article in 1951. Most of his patients were athletes in their teens or twenties, some professional. The majority referred to the chronic injury as a "weak or trick" ankle. Running and particularly cutting caused a painful snapping sensation anterior to the lateral malleolus radiating to the head of the fibula. A click was often heard. Compression of the fibula against the talus caused pain and swelling. These signs and symptoms were due to the pinching of a large soft tissue mass at the talofibular articulation. The meniscoid was noted in sprains only by Wolin[6], but should be suspected in undisplaced fibular fractures.

X-rays are usually negative or show some ossification of the fibular collateral ligament caused by partial disruption or hematoma formation plus subsequent tissue organization. There is sometimes a spur at the anterior lip of the talus. Stress films at times show a tilting of the talus due to the rupture (usually partial) of the anterior talofibular ligament and capsule. The majority of cases, however, do not show any significant instability.

All failed to respond to conservative treatment. Originally, open excision was required before the advent of arthroscopy. The cases reported by the above author (Wolin)[6] showed dramatic relief with this treatment. At present, excision can be performed arthroscopically, employing mechanical distraction, as described for the synovial impingement lesions. This also allows further exploration of the ankle joint by superior techniques.

Results are expected to be equally as good with less morbidity and rehabilitation. Further experience will clarify the relationship of these pathological soft tissue lesions.

Posterior Soft Tissue Impingement

There are three (and possibly four) types of potential soft tissue posterior impingement lesions that may occur, as recognized at the time of this writing, other than chronic synovitis, adhesions, and the extension of the lateral synovial impingement. They may be responsible for symptoms in the posterior ankle or area of the hindfoot and should be amenable to arthroscopic diagnosis and excision. These additional lesions are the hypertrophied transverse tibiofibular ligament (and/or tibial slip), meniscus of the ankle, and a pathological labrum of the posterior ankle joint.

The first structure is the transverse tibiofibular ligament. A similar structure was referred to by Chen[4] and Ikeuchi[3] as the posterior or tibial slip. According to the author's investigation, these may at times be one and the same structure or exist as separate entities. If they exist as double structures, the transverse tibiofibular ligament is most likely the lesion of concern. According to Harty,[7] variations, such as mentioned here, occur in the ankle joint. This manifestation was also noted arthroscopically in the knee and other joints in the past. The author has limited arthroscopic surgery experience with these entities except for three cases of the hypertrophied transverse tibiofibular ligament. One of these was clearly considered to be pathological, and the only cause or explanation of the chronic pain. Therefore, these structures or lesions merit discussion in this text.

The transverse tibiofibular ligaments (and/or tibial slips) vary considerably in size and may appear as large adhesions if not properly identified, especially by the inexperienced arthroscopist. This may be because of its variation in size, structure and position in relationship to the synovial lining of the posterior ankle joint. It lies posterior or behind the synovial membrane, appears quite small and inconspicuous on some occasions and at other times is enlarged or markedly hypertrophied (or a double structure). These structures may receive more attention with the increasing interest in arthroscopy of the ankle and the advent of mechanical distraction.

Anatomically, the transverse tibiofibular ligament runs in an oblique fashion from its distal fibular origin (adjacent to and proximal to the origin of the posterior talofibular ligament) to the posterior tibia at the junction of the medial malleolus (Figure 9-16). It is just beneath the posterior tibiofibular ligament. Chen[4] and Ikeuchi,[3] as stated, mentioned a "posterior or tibial slip" and described it as originating from the posterior talofibular ligament itself and running to the posterior tibia. Chen[4] has reported this entity as resulting in fibrosis because of trauma to the ankle. The author has observed the transverse tibiofibular ligament to be an anatomical structure with which one must now become familiar when performing arthroscopy of the ankle. Additionally, on at least one occasion, as stated, when enlarged and hypertrophied, it is a pathological entity. A distinction should be made as to whether it should be partially excised or not (Figures 9-17 and 9-18).

Hamilton[5] reported another distinct structure seen in the posterior ankle joint in ballet dancers, which he referred to as a "meniscus of the ankle." There have been cases that would present with a tear such as a bucket handle lesion, which would displace into the joint and become symptomatic. Further study confirmed that a meniscus type of structure, exists in some patients similar in location to that found in certain marsupials, such as the kangaroo. This entity, when seen in man, also histologically proves to be a true meniscus. The clinical signs and symptoms, according to Myerson,[8] are pain and tenderness in the posterior ankle and hindfoot, just anterior to the usual location of a retrocalcaneal bursitis. The pain is aggravated by descending stairs. He has diagnosed this lesion by MR, prior to arthroscopic excision (Figures 9-19 and 9-20). Again, this needs further study, but appears to be of practical application in cases of unsubstantiated pain in the posterior ankle and hindfoot.

Also, a labrum of the posterior lip of the tibia was seen and discussed by Hamilton. This occurs on infrequent occasions in the human ankle. When injured, the tibial labrum can become pathological just like its counterpart in the shoulder joint.

Chen[4] has reported that he views hypertrophy of the posterior talofibular ligament as the cause of local chronic pain. Whether this will be amenable to partial arthroscopic excision remains to be proven by further arthroscopic study.

All of the lesions can be the source of the posterior soft tissue impingement and subject to consideration in the differential diagnosis (Chapter VIII) of ankle pain. In addition, other nonsoft tissue lesions of the posterior ankle compartment can occur other than chondral and osteochondral loose bodies. These are the enlarged posterior tibial lip and a nonunited posterior talar facet (Parks[11]). Open surgery in those latter two entities would most likely be necessary. Arthroscopic excision of the soft tissue lesions with the use of distraction now appears to be the procedure of choice. Any combination of portals (described in Chapter XVI) may be employed for triangulation in the posterior ankle joint.

Infectious Synovitis

Infectious synovitis or septic arthritis of the ankle has been proven to be amenable to arthroscopic treatment. This would normally be expected since the value of arthroscopic surgery in the acute and chronic septic knee has been shown. The author has seen one such ankle case that will be described and which has responded dramatically to arthroscopic intervention. In advanced cases, ingress and egress tubes can be placed arthroscopically for adequate irrigation and drainage (Schonholtz).[31]

Case Reviews

Case 1. C.V. Local Synovitis

This 37-year-old man was seen by the author for pain on the lateral aspect of the left ankle for eight months aggravated by sport activities. There was no history of injury. A bone scan had been done and was negative. Examination showed pain on inverting the ankle. The pain was located laterally and there was local tenderness of 1+ degree. Motion and stability were good, and there was no swelling. Routine x-rays were negative. Conservative treatment consisted of antiinflammatory medications, physical therapy, and an injection of a steroid with no relief. An arthroscopic examination was performed with the use of the distraction device for the first time. A prominent mass of synovial tissue, a few adhesions, and capsule-appearing tissue were seen and removed from the lateral talomalleolar joint. Immediate relief was seen at the first postoperative visit and was sustained to date two years later. The patient was happy and felt that he was 70% improved. He was able to return to his regular recreational athletic activities which included running, swimming, and volleyball. Prior to surgery he was completely curtailed from sports.

Case 2. J.K. Synovial Impingement Syndrome and Chondral Defect

This 42-year-old man was seen for intermittent pain located medially and laterally in the ankle joint. This pain resulted from a twisting injury which he received playing tennis several months earlier. He also complained of "giving way". Examination showed minimal tenderness medially and laterally. There was slight swelling about the lateral malleolus. Motion was good, despite guarding. AP stress films showed a talotibial angle of seven to eight degress (also the same postoperatively), slightly more than the opposite side. A bone scan showed a minimal increased uptake of the right talus. Both a tomogram and arthrogram were negative.

Arthroscopic examination with distraction was done and showed a large area of thick and inflamed synovial tissue at the junction of the fibula and plafond (lateral talomalleolar joint recess), and also attached to the undersurface of the interosseous membrane. Pigmentation was seen on the surface of this lesion. The same tissue extended posteriorly, around the peroneal tendons, and to the medial talomalleolar joint, but to a much lesser degree. Examination of the articular cartilage showed a loose area on the medial side of the midtalar dome. The loose articular cartilage was easily lifted off with a probe. The underlying lesions were locally debrided, abraded to bleeding bone, and drilled.

Tissue was removed in the usual manner. The pathology slides showed gray-white to gray-tan multiple fragments, soft to moderately resilient. Histologically, synovial lining cells with increased prominence and mild synovial hyperplasia was apparent. The articular cartilage showed an unremarkable lacunar pattern.

Postoperatively, the patient was relieved immediately, although not completely. There was some persistent slight aching, apparently because of the abraded area. This gradually subsided with time as the area filled in with good fibrocartilagenous tissue. Weight bearing was restricted for only a few weeks. Followup one-and-a-half years later showed significant improvement maintained.

The bone scan, stress films, and the nature of the injury by history would explain the cartilage defect (with minimal bone) associated with the synovial impingement lesions (Figures 9-21 and 9-22).

Case 3. C.S. Soft Tissue Pathology (Posterolateral Lesion) (Ganglion, Nodule)

This 16-year-old girl was seen for pain in the ankle joint of 4 months duration. It gradually increased and persisted. This disabled her, causing her difficulty in walking and performing her usual activities. There was crepitus and swelling, combined with the pain. The pain was generalized at first, but then became localized over the lateral aspect of the ankle and deep within the joint. She would often stand on the outside of her foot to gain some momentary relief. Unsuccessful conservative treatment was followed by an arthroscopic examination by her referring orthopedic surgeon. This exam was reported as negative at that time. Still the symptoms persisted. When seen by the author, initial examination showed minimal swelling, guarding, and minimal restriction of flexion and extension of about ten degrees. The ankle was both clinically stable and stable with stress films. An arthrogram was reported as negative. She had an arthroscopic examination with the distraction device. Synovial debridement of the anterior ankle joint compartment had to be done for visualization. Initially, the lesion could not be found. Further distention, distraction, and probing were employed. A tough elastic fibrosed synovial tissue cystic mass about the size of a small grape was found in the extreme posterolateral aspect of the joint. This structure was adjacent to the peroneal tendons and when probed would slip in and out of the joint (ganglion of tenosynovial sheath).

The anterolateral approach and the central approach were used for ease of examination and treatment. As the ganglion was removed with a basket forceps, much more such tissue was pulled from areas adjacent to the joint and from above the joint line. The lesion was much larger than when first seen. Further impingement occurred when distraction was disengaged momentarily. Complete removal was performed with the motorized shaver and cutter. Pathological examination showed gray-white, yellow-tan, free, firm tissue. Microscopic section showed fibrous tissue and partially hyalinized connective tissue. Papillary projections of synovial tissue were blunt and covered by thickened proliferating synovial cells. The patient was relieved immediately and remained so until the time of this writing. She resumed all previous sport activities (Figure 9-23).

Case 4. D.L. Adhesions

This 37-year-old woman was seen by the author for symptoms following an undisplaced fracture of the distal tibia that occurred nine months before. Her leg was casted appropriately, but after healing was complete there was recurrent pain, popping, and instability. She had injections, ankle supports, and ultrasound without relief. Examination showed ten degrees limitation of extension, pain in the inner aspect with inversion, less on eversion, minimal generalized swelling and multiple tender areas. The ankle was stable clinically and on x-rays. She then had an arthroscopic examination with the distraction device. Numerous thick adhesions were noted throughout the joint with coexisting chronic reactive synovitis. A large adhesion created a groove along the anterior dome of the talus accounting for the clicking, popping, and a feeling of recurrent instability. The adhesions were excised and an arthroscopic synovectomy was performed. The pathology exam showed microscopically a pinkish-gray soft tissue. When viewed microscopically, the synovium showed nonspecific nodular and villus hyperplasia. Complete relief was obtained for two months following this procedure. She then had minimal symptoms but good relief with an arch support. The patient felt that she was about 60% improved. The swelling remained reduced, but she still noted occasional stiffness and mild clicking. Further treatment was declined, and she stated that she was satisfied with her result.

Experience observed with this case and others, indicated that with preventative measures and improved postoperative care, a better result might have been obtained. Therefore, instillation of epinephrine (0.5% Marcaine with epinephrine 1 to 200,000) at the conclusion of the surgery, elevation, ice packing of the ankle and postoperative aspirations when necessary are now recommended. This should be followed by early motion, stretching, and strengthening exercises. In the future, it would seem reasonable to warn patients about recurrence when adhesions are suspected. On such occasions, the procedure may have to be repeated (Figures 9-24 and 9-25).

Case 5. W.C. Synovial Chondromatosis

This 17-year-old boy was seen by the author for a long history of generalized aching pain in the ankle joint that was aggravated by strenuous activity. This particularly bothered him during athletics. The aching would increase, and be accompanied by swelling after participation in any sport. The physical findings were minimal swelling and generalized pain on manipulating the ankle. Motion was slightly limited in all directions. The original x-rays were not remarkable. An arthrogram and a CT scan were forwarded by the referring orthopedic surgeon and showed this to be a fairly obvious case of synovial chondromatosis. It is interesting to note that most of the loose bodies were located in the posterolateral aspect of the ankle joint.

Mechanical distraction was particularly helpful in treatment, considering the location of the lesions. The arthroscopic examination showed multiple small loose bodies. Some of these were suctioned from the joint, and others were flushed or pulled from the posterior compartment to the anterior joint with a probe. The larger ones were grasped and removed. At the conclusion, a limited synovectomy was done. The patient was on crutches and wore a short, light cast for about three weeks. After this he underwent a period of rehabilitation under the direction of the referring orthopedic surgeon. He rapidly returned to normal activity and had no more symptoms. A year later it was learned that he had completed a successful senior year of high school football and had been recruited to a major college football team (Figures 9-26 through 9-30).

Case 6. M.A. Infectious Synovitis

This 15-year-old boy had a rather severe ankle sprain while playing football. He was treated by repeated casting. Months later he continued to have recurrent pain on several occasions. After a repeat episode, the patient was seen by the author for the first time. He presented with acute severe pain, tenderness, and swelling in the ankle joint. Following a complete clinical evaluation, a bone scan was done and showed an extensive radioactive uptake. Fifteen ccs of purulent material was aspirated from an acutely tender ankle.

Response to arthroscopic debridement and antibiotics was dramatic, the temperature fell immediately, and recovery was complete. There was no damage to the articular cartilage. He was rapidly rehabilitated and back to normal activity within about eight weeks (Figures 9-31 through 9-34).

Discussion

This study of soft tissue impingement lesions was not done to statistically or scientifically document results, but to establish their existence as a significant pathological entity. As mentioned previously, long term followup of a prospective series is not possible until adequate time has elapsed. The purpose here is to show the need for arthroscopic surgery of this entity, indicate the general response to treatment, as of this date, and make appropriate recommendations. The facts necessary to accomplish this end were tabulated in Tables 9-1, 9-2, and 9-3.

It is of importance to note that 23 of the 29 patients were referred by 14 orthopedic surgeons and by four family practice physicians. The duration of symptoms noted, disability, and lack of response to conservative measures are clear indications as to patients' need for arthroscopic intervention. Information was obtained on all but one patient who was lost to followup. Fourteen of these patients were examined by the author and the remainder had to be interviewed by phone since they lived outside of the area. No patients were classified as excellent because of the short term of the study and by the authors choice, although several of them said they were in that category. A few patients were downgraded because of recurrent symptoms but responded to subsequent conservative treatment. One patient returned to athletics prematurely and had a temporary setback. Clinical exam suggested (and an MRI substantiated) a tendinitis of the common extensor tendon (Figure 9-35). Further successful treatment was accomplished with open surgical exploration and debridement.

Also, it should be kept in mind that there was coexisting pathology and, in some cases, litigation that might affect results. These patients were not upgraded for that reason, and the end result was accepted.

In summary, all but four patients were satisfied and 25 of the 28 were significantly improved. As a result of this experience, recommendations are considered appropriate for the purpose of improving the care of future patients:

1. Select patients properly.
2. Do an adequate preoperative clinical and x-ray evaluation (Chapter III).
3. Anticipate preoperatively or recognize at surgery coexisting lesions and give the patient an appropriate prognosis.
4. Evaluate the impingement in its entirety.
5. Do an adequate excision of all impingement tissue and treat associated pathology.
6. Employ proper postoperative care, physical therapy, and rehabilitation (Chapter XV).

Table 9-1.
Followup Study

Referring Source.
- Orthopedic Surgeon. 14 (23 patients)
- Family Physician. 4 (4 patients)
- Nonreferral. (1 patient)

Average Duration
of Symptoms. 23 months (range 22 to 17 years)

Preoperative Conservative Treatment.	Yes (19)	No (8)	Unknown (1)

Pathology.
- Local Chronic Synovitis. 1
- Lateral Impingement Lesion. 15
- Medial Impingement Lesion. 1
- Medial and Lateral Lesions. 1
- Posterolateral Lesion. 6
- Posterior Impingement. 1 (TT FL or tibial slip)
- Meniscoid. 2

Table 9-2.
Followup Study

Associated Pathology.
- Plafond Defect. 1
- Dome Defect. 2
- Chondromalacia. 1
- Degenerative Arthritis. 1
- Loose Body. 1
- Previous Reconstruction. 4
- Osteophyte. 2
- Neuroma and Reflex Dystrophy. 1
- Tendinitis E.D.C. 1

Followup.
- Average 8 months (range 2 to 23 months)

Other Factors.
- Legal. 3
- Compensation. 6

Table 9-3.
Followup Study

Result.
- Satisfied. 24
- Not Satisfied. 4
- Improved. 25
- Good. 16
- Fair. 9
- Poor. 3

Subsequent Treatment.
- Hardware Removed. 2
- Physical Therapy. 2
- Injection (Arthroscopic incision). 2
- Infected Incisional Site. 1
- Debridement EDC Tendon. 1

References
1. Schonholtz GJ: Arthroscopic Surgery of the Shoulder, Elbow And Ankle. Springfield, IL. Charles C. Thomas. 1986.
2. Beltran J, Noto AM, Mosure JC, et al: Ankle: Surface Coil MR Imaging At 1.5 Tl. Rad 161:203-209, 1986.
3. Ikeuchi H: Personal Communication.
4. Chen Y: Arthroscopy Of The Ankle Joint. In: Arthroscopy Of Small Joints. Watanabe M., New York, IGAKU-SHOIN, 1985.
5. Hamilton W.G. and Sheskier S: The Marsupial Meniscus As A Course Of Posterior Impingement In Dancers. In preparation for Foot & Ankle.
6. Wolin I, Glassman F, Sideman S, et al: Internal Derangement Of Talofibular Components Of The Ankle. Surg Gyn & Ob 91:193-200, 1950.
7. Harty M: Personal Communication, 1986.
8. Myerson M: Personal Communication, 1986.
9. Ferkle R: Personal Communication, 1987.
10. Menbenbaum BR: Person Communication, 1987.
11. Parks JC: Injuries of the Hindfoot Clinical Orthopedics 122: 28-36, Jan 1977.

CHAPTER 10

OSTEOCHONDRITIS DISSECANS

James F. Guhl, M.D.

Osteochondritis dissecans is synonymous with osteochondral fracture of the dome of the talus, and is also referred to as a transcondylar fracture, interarticular fracture, or a flake fracture.

A review of the theories regarding the etiology and early treatment of this entity will be presented. Emphasis is placed on a study of the scientific articles from the late 19th century until the prearthroscopic era. Concepts regarding pathology and the results of treating osteochondritis dissecans to that time are evaluated. With this in mind, the impact of diagnostic arthroscopy and arthroscopic surgery of the ankle during the early 1980s is noted. Established ideas have been subject to change, causing the need to update our understanding of this lesion of the ankle joint.

Etiology

In 1856, Alexander Munro[15] described loose bodies in the ankle joint for the first time. Konig[12] in 1888 classified loose bodies in other joints and explained spontaneous necrosis as their origin. He originated the term osteochondritis dissecans. Barth[4] described the same lesion in 1898, and explained it as an interarticular fracture with or without trauma. Fisher[9] in 1920 and Phemister[26] in 1924 classified the many conditions producing loose bodies. Kappis[11] in 1922 was the first to use the term osteochondritis of the ankle joint. In 1932, Rendu[21] described it as an interarticular fracture of the talus. Brendt and Harty[3] reviewed the world literature in 1959, and presented their own theories. They suggested the term "transchondral fracture" of the talus and determined that this best described the lesion both etiologically and pathologically. O'Donoghue,[17] in the mid-1960s also stated that these lesions were interarticular fractures.

Davidson et al.[8] felt that although O'Donoghue's[17] work referred primarily to the knee joint, it also applied to any discussions of the ankle joint. In 1956, in a separate discussion, Goldstone and Pisani,[10] as well as Campbell and Ranawat[6] indicated that there were other causes than trauma for the etiology of osteochondritis dissecans of the ankle. Campbell and Ranawat[6] pointed out that bone infarction preceded these pathological fractures.

The predominant theory regarding etiology, however still appeared to be trauma. Yvars,[25] in 1976, Alexander and Lichtman[1] in 1979, and others later in their clinical series, emphasized that the etiology was trauma and the treatment was operative. In Canale's[7] series of 1981, 25 of 29 injuries were due to trauma. Since the days of Brendt and Harty,[3] trauma has been considered the leading cause of osteochondritis dissecans or osteochondral fractures.

Incidence

Osteochondritis of the talus comprises about 4% of all cases of osteochondritis dissecans. The age group in most series is between about 20 to 30 years for most patients. McCullough and Venugopal[14] reported an average age of 27 years in their series. Males predominate slightly in most series reported.

Medial dome lesions are more common in most series than lateral lesions. Yao and Weis[24] reported 56 lesions located on the medial aspect of the talar dome, as compared to 43 of the lateral talar dome. In reviewing several series, the incidence of bilateral lesions averages about 10%. According to Brendt and Harty,[3] nine of 207 cases were bilateral. Blum and Strijk[5] reported that two of 16 were bilateral in their study. Lindholm, Osterman, and Vankka[13] stated that three of 17 were bilateral. There were two central lesions in Canales'[7] series of 29.

Mechanism of Injury

According to Yao and Weis,[24] lateral lesions are thought to be caused by eversion of the foot with the ankle dorsiflexed and the tibia internally rotated on the talus. These lesions are almost always secondary to trauma. The medial lesions are apparently caused by inversion of the foot with the ankle plantar flexed. They may occur, however, without any preceding trauma.

Location

Lesions of the medial aspect of the dome of the talus occur in the mid or posterior third. Osteochondral fractures on the lateral side of the dome are in the mid or anterior portion (with exceptions) (Figure 10-1).

Structural Characteristics

Medial dome lesions are usually asymmetrical while lateral dome lesions are symmetrical. Also the medial lesions appear to be deep, cup shaped and usually remain in situ. The lateral lesions are more shallow. Medial lesions have fewer symptoms, heal spontaneously at times, and do not cause development of arthritis, according to Cannale.[7] According to Rodin,[22] lateral lesions rarely heal (with conservative treatment), cause more symptoms, and, sometimes, early arthritic changes develop after open surgery.

Stage

According to Brendt and Harty,[3] lesions of the talar dome were staged as to their appearance at surgery. Stage I was defined as a compression fracture without displacement (intact). Stage II represented an incomplete avulsion of the osteochondral fragment (early separation). Stage III was complete avulsion of an osteochondral fragment without displacement (separated). Stage IV was a completely displaced osteochondral fragment (displaced). The latter often lies upside down in the crater or may be completely separated from the lesion. This classification applies to both medial and lateral lesions (Figures 10-2 through 10-4).

Brendt and Harty[3] concluded in 1959, and Cannale[7] agreed, that Stage I and II lesions, medial or lateral, should be treated with nonoperative measures, as well as Stage III medial lesions. Lateral Stage III and medial and lateral Stage IV lesions should have immediate excision of the fragment and curettage. Blum and Strijk[6] stated that it was their experience that the difference between Stage II and Stage III was not always distinguished by -ray techniques. They also stated that the degree of involvement of bone and cartilage can vary from fracture of only the cartilage (i.e., chondral fracture) to fracture of only the osseous part, which leaves the lining cartilage intact (the latter was expressed by Brendt and Harty[3] as a transchondral fracture).

Both medial and lateral lesions can predispose to the formation of loose bodies, more so in the latter.

It is important to appreciate that the arthroscopic evaluation has altered the interpretation of the x-ray classification of osteochondritis diseases. This will be demonstrated in the case review and summarized in the conclusion of this chapter.

Conservative Versus Surgical Treatment

Since the classical report of Brendt and Harty[3] in 1959, surgical treatment has been considered superior to conservative care (with few exceptions). Several series were cited to support this claim. Acromonano et al.[2] did treat some patients conservatively, if the arthrogram showed no break in the articular cartilage of the talus. McCollough and Venugopal[14] recommended two months of conservative treatment and then surgical treatment if symptoms continued. In general, lesions in situ were treated nonoperatively. From 1959 to the present time, surgeons followed the indications for operative treatment based on the Brendt and Harty[3] classification, and recommended further by Cannale and Belding.[7] Other series emphasizing surgical treatment are those of Blom and Strijk[5] in 1975, Yvars[25] in 1975, Alexander and Lichtman[1] in 1979, and O'Farrell and Costello in 1982.[18]

Drilling the Base

Drilling the base of the reconstructed lesion has been almost uniformly recommended in all series during the last 25 years. Yvars:[25] "Drilling is important in excised lesions." Scharling:[23] "In all cases, drilling was done into the site of osteochondritis or through the cysts, except in one case in which a cyst was filled with bone chips." O'Farrell and Costello:[18] "Of the 15 patients with good results, 12 had had drilling of the base of the defect. Of the nine patients with fair results, only two of them had drilling of the defect. Drilling of the base of the defect should always be performed after excision of the osteochondritic fragment." Alexander and Lichtman:[1] "The surgical treatment consists of drilling and curettage followed by nonweight bearing and early range of motion exercises. We used fine curettes to excise the lesion. Then the base of the cartilage defect was scraped and drilled with small drill points to encourage fibrocartilagenous filling of the defect." O'Donoghue[17] in his 1966 classic publication in the *Journal of Traumatology* strongly recommended drilling of the base of the crater after excision of the fragments.

Malleolar Osteotomy

Some authors stated that medial malleolar osteotomy was harmless in the treatment of osteochondritis dissecans (Scharling, O'Farrell, and Costello). O'Farrell and Costello,[18] however, did have one nonunion out of eight medial malleolar osteotomies done to gain access to the lesions of the medial talar dome.

McCullough and Venugopal:[14] "An anterolateral approach provides good exposure for surgical treatment of the lateral lesion, while osteotomy of the medial malleolus is usually necessary for medial lesions. This is a further insult to the ankle and may in itself be a contributory factor to the subsequent development of osteoarthritis."

It has been the author's experience in his practice over the past 25 years that an increased morbidity is often noted with the performance of a medial malleolar osteotomy. In one such case, pain persisted at the osteotomy site long after healing of the lesion. Obviously, with arthroscopic treatment, this and the open operation can now be avoided.

Postoperative Care

The standards of postoperative care will change with the addition of arthroscopic treatment of osteochondritis dissecans. Yvars[25] stated that early resumption of motion and weight bearing is recommended at two weeks postoperatively, if no osteotomy is done. Alexander and Lichtman[1] advised a cast for seven to ten days with no weight bearing, followed by early range of motion and strengthening exercises. This would be continued eight to twelve weeks if there were an osteotomy done. In general, if an osteotomy were necessary, casting was recommended eight to twelve weeks, followed by exercises and then later weight bearing, as tolerated.

The author has had several patients begin weight bearing a few weeks after an arthroscopic reconstruction, which consisted of excision, debridement, abrasion, and drilling. Good results followed this regime.

Healing on X-Ray

Healing may be difficult, and, at times, impossible to determine by x-ray studies. In the author's experience, almost half of the lesions showed little evidence of healing, or little change on x-ray, long after clinical healing had occurred. There are some techniques that are of help. Followup x-rays taken by the same technique that originally showed the lesion best preoperatively will help in determining healing. Lateral lesions located anteriorly, which are best seen on mortise views with dorsiflexion, should be followed during healing with that viewing technique. Medial lesions, most often located posteriorly, should be followed by views in plantar flexion. Tomograms which show the trabecular pattern in greater detail are a superior means of determining healing. Magnification views should also be considered for this purpose. Bone scans have been found to be of no help.

Analysis of Results

Prearthroscopic Era

Rsults were better in most series with operative treatment, except in a few cases where the indications for conservative treatment were well defined. In the series reported below this was further emphasized. Blom and Strijk[5] stated that operative treatment gave better results than in patients treated conservatively. This was true for medial and lateral lesions. Brendt and Harty[3] stated: "Of 149 patients treated nonsurgically, 73.9% were poor, 8.7% fair, and only 17.4% good. Of 56 surgically treated patients, 73.6% had good results." However, there was considerable variation in conservative treatment in the latter series. This affected the results reported above to a significant degree. Naumetz and Schweigal[16] reported that the results of 31 cases, which failed to respond to conservative treatment, later had the lesions excised, debrided, curetted, and drilled. The results were 63% good, 30% fair, and 7% poor. O'Farrell and Costello[18] stated that in their series of 24 surgically excised osteochondritis dissecans lesion cases with a four year followup there were 15 good, nine fair and one poor result. They concluded that early surgery, done before 12 months from the time of onset (or injury), gave the best results.

Alexander and Lichtman,[1] in their 25 patient series, with an average followup of 65 months, reported 88% good results. These four series, at best, averaged 71% good results with surgery (during the prearthroscopic era). Canale and Belding[7] reviewed 24 cases of talar osteochondritis dissecans initially treated with immobilization in short leg casts or a PT brace for 12 to 18 weeks. Fifteen patients required surgery after symptoms persisted for more than six months. On comparing the stage and site of the lesion with results of treatment, they agreed with Brendt and Harty's recommendation.

Arthroscopic Era

With arthroscopy, the classification and subsequent treatment of osteochondritis dissecans will change. Based on the author's 12 cases including those discussed, there is reason to expect a significant percentage of improvement of results in the future.

Case Reviews

Intact Lesions

Case 1 R.M. For clinical history, please see the captions to Figures 10-5 through 10-10.

Case 2 M.K. (Figures 10-11 and 10-12). This 19-year-old girl was seen for pain in the right ankle that had been persistent for eight months. There was no trauma, and it was getting progressively worse, with difficulty in walking. Examination showed tenderness medially with pain in the area aggravated by plantar flexion. X-rays, including tomograms, showed a lucent defect in the posterior medial aspect of the dome of the talus. There was also a small bone fragment within the lesion, but no sclerotic base. The bone scan was positive with moderate uptake. Arthroscopy with distraction was performed and showed no evidence of a lesion either by probing or viewing the talar dome. The area of the lesion was drilled by the transmalleolar approach with an .062 Kirschner wire. The extremity was then immobilized in plaster for nine weeks and the patient progressed to full weight bearing. She improved fully and in six months was satisfied. The patient rated herself a seven on a scale of zero to ten at the time of this writing, since then she had some difficulty when running. X-ray showed the nidus was still quite visible in this clinically healed intact lesion.

This is an example of an intact lesion as seen at arthroscopy. However, it appeared on x-ray examination to be separated. This example is the opposite of case 2 and case 3. It is also an example of a lesion persisting on x-ray long after clinical healing occurred.

Case 3 J.P. Early Separation (Figures 10-13 and 10-14). This 15-year-old girl injured her right ankle while running track. She was seen six months later for persistent pain and guarding in the posterolateral aspect of that joint. X-rays showed a radiolucent area, seen best in the mortise view. This was located in the anterolateral aspect of the dome of the talus. The bone scan was positive. Lateral tomograms further defined the lesion and showed that it was no larger than seen in the regular x-rays and there was no sclerotic base or nidus. The diagnosis therefore was an "intact" osteochondritis dissecans. Arthroscopic examination (and surgery) were done with the distraction method.

Faint, white, softened articular cartilage was found on the lateral dome, surrounded by pale, yellow, glistening normal appearing articular cartilage. There was only a little difference in color, no change in the contour, and no apparent break in the articular cartilage. There was also no elevation or depression. With the use of a probe, the affected cartilage was easily lifted off of the lesion, indicating that there was early separation. Reconstruction (debridement, abrasion, and drilling) of the defect was then done arthroscopically. Postoperatively, she was placed in an ankle immobilizer for two weeks and remained nonweightbearing for three weeks postoperatively. The patient gradually improved and was kept out of sports for the rest of the school year. At the time of this writing (over two years later) she has remained asympotomatic. The lesion receded on x-ray.

Case 4 J.G. (Figures 10-15 through 10-18). This 30-year-old man was seen by the author for continued ankle pain. He had injured his right ankle playing basketball ten months previous to presentation. There were persistent symptoms and a lesion was seen on x-ray consistent with an osteochondral defect of the talar dome. He had an arthroscopic examination done by the referring orthopedic surgeon three months postinjury. At that time, distraction was not used. There were no notable pathological findings. A minimal debridement was done. After surgery, symptoms persisted with pain and swelling. The pain was aggravated by plantar flexion and inversion. X-rays then showed a faint lesion with a minimal ill sclerotic border (seen best in the oblique x-rays and tomograms). No nidus or loose body was noted. The size of the lesion was the same by tomogram as by x-ray. At surgery, with distraction, the talar dome appeared normal. When probed, there was a soft, resilient area with very slight discoloration on the lateral aspect of the talus. The articular cartilage had no apparent break on the surface, but the area described above became easily detached with a probe, again indicating early separation. A reconstruction consisting of trimming, debridement, abrasion, and drilling of the base was done. Postoperative active motion was begun one week after surgery. The advice of nonweight bearing walking with crutches for three weeks was followed by the patient. The patient remains improved at two years.

Case 5 R.R. Separated Lesion (Figures 10-19 through 10-22). This 25-year-old woman was seen with intermittent pain in her ankle for five years. The symptoms became worse during the final two months of that period. There was a sensation of cracking and buckling, with pain and tenderness, noted on the medial side of the joint. Dorsiflexion was limited by ten degrees. She had difficulty performing her job as a flight attendent, particularly when she had to wear high heels. The x-rays showed a large defect, 1cm by 2cm in diameter, with a sclerotic border in the medial talus. The lesion was located slightly posterior. Tomograms showed a definite nidus within the lesion. At arthroscopy, with distraction, there was a large fragment at the base of the lesion that was completely separated. The fragment was removed, and the base of the lesion debrided, abraded, and drilled. The patient began immediate motion after surgery, and was weight bearing two weeks later. She was relatively asymptomatic in three weeks, and back to work as a flight attendant in six weeks. Several months later, when seen again, she remained asymptomatic, even though wearing high heels. She was satisfied and rated herself an eight on a scale of zero to ten at one year. Clinical examination showed no significant findings, except for the healed incisions. X-rays showed that the lesion was fainter than prior to surgery, but still present.

Case 6 E.E. Salvaged Case (Figures 10-23 through 10-28). This 37-year-old man was seen with a history of pain in the right ankle for two years. The referring orthopedic surgeon had done an arthrotomy and curettage two years prior, with removal of a loose body. Drilling was not done at that time. When examined by this author, review of the x-rays showed a large lesion persisted. A CT scan showed that it was even more extensive than on x-ray. A bone scan showed the lesion of the right ankle had considerable uptake, but there was also an area of weak response in the left ankle. Several x-rays finally showed a small lesion in that ankle that was asymptomatic and therefore not treated at that time.

At arthroscopy, with distraction of the right ankle, the crater was seen filled with fibrocartilage that appeared to be of poor quality. When this was probed, a large flap was easily developed. Complete debridement was then done and revealed that the lesion was larger than expected, according to the x-ray, and did confirm the findings of the CT scan. Reconstruction, including drilling, was done at the base of the lesion and into the posterior aspect of the crater, where the remainder of the lesion was located beneath good articular cartilage. It was advised that the patient should remain nonweight bearing for approximately ten weeks due to the large size of the lesion and because it was a second procedure. Range of motion exercises were started with crutch walking a week following surgery. The patient remained improved one and one-half years later. The left ankle was done in a simpler fashion, and a second look at the right ankle showed good fibrocartilagenous healing.

A detailed report of results is not considered appropriate at present for this text. However, experience noted in these cases, and with six others in this series (and eight subsequent cases) indicate that one might expect a better response utilizing these arthroscopic techniques. Certainly, the previously indicated need for arthrotomy and medial malleolar osteotomy has been eliminated. It also appears that early weight bearing has been established as a result of this study (cases 3, 4, 5, and others).

Analysis: Osteochondritis Dissecans

Arthroscopic Era

The introduction of arthroscopy for the diagnosis and treatment of osteochondritis dissecans and dome fractures of the talus appears to give hope of improved results regarding these pathological entities. Mechanical distraction should add another valuable tool in surgery performed for these lesions. Prior to this, the exact status of the health of the articular cartilage could not always be evaluated as well. However now, direct viewing and probing is better accomplished. The value of the posterolateral portal is shown in Figures 10-31 through 10-36 (and others). While the x-rays may have suggested that the lesion was intact, direct observation often proved otherwise, and would therefore affect treatment and prognosis. Admittedly, tomograms, arthrograms, and CT scans add information. Nothing, however, can compare with direct visualization and probing for accurate classification.

This reclassification has better indicated the surgical techniques required. For example, intact lesions as found on x-ray have at times been seen to be separated at arthroscopy, and lesions that appeared separated were subsequently found to be intact. Furthermore, intact lesions in young patients can now be treated by arthroscopic drilling (transmolleolor), in addition to, or instead of, casting alone.

While these gains appear evident, it must be recognized that the bone scan has been most helpful in the discovery of lesions not seen on routine and special x-ray views. Use of CT scans has further defined their location and extent (more so than tomograms). Finally, MR imagery has revealed some lesions not seen by any other method. (See Chapter IV and Figures 3-24 through 3-27.)

With the advent of arthroscopy and distraction, it has been often seen that the articular cartilage is a little soft or fibrillated, and, therefore, will invariably become loose with time. Areas of elevation and depression are often observed. Small areas of the border where fibrous tissue may protrude is observed on occasion. If the above changes are present, there is no reason to try to save the cartilage or separated osteochondral fragments. These pathological changes are irreversible and healing in situ cannot be expected. Further observations dictate that the treatment should be removal of the loose cartilage or fragments, and curetting, abrading, and drilling the base to freshly bleeding bone.

CT scans can be used along with direct observation arthroscopically to determine the extent of the lesion. There may be a small area of diseased articular cartilage overlying a large area of necrotic bone (as seen in case 5). The necrotic bone portion of the lesion is usually more posterior and deep to the healthy osteocartilagenous covering. Therefore, drilling in a posterior direction from the area or crater that has been reconstructed should be considered, as well as drilling from above through the healthy osteochondral layer into necrotic bone, and into freshly bleeding bone below, to stimulate revascularization.

The goal of treatment is to obtain good, tough fibrocartilagenous tissue to fill the defect. This will yield the best results. Treatment other than reconstruction (excision, debridement, abrading, and drilling) is very likely to lead to degenerative arthritis at an early age, in the author's opinion.

"Stage I lesions," as seen on x-ray, should not be treated conservatively, if at arthroscopy there is unhealthy articular cartilage. This practice may suffice temporarily, causing a remission for a few years, but, ultimately, the chondral surface will break down and the lesion will not heal. For this reason, all talar lesions of osteochondritis dissecans should be arthroscoped. In addition to better evaluation and subsequent treatment, the arthroscope with distraction allows more accurate surgery, since this is done, with more room under magnification with appropriate instruments and television monitoring.

Transmalleolar surgery with distraction for drilling the base of reconstructed lesions is preferred, rather than an arthrotomy and osteotomy, for the reconstruction and drilling. The intact lesion in young patients confirmed at arthroscopic examination should also be treated with transmalleolar drilling for revascularization. This is another advantage of arthroscopy over cast treatment alone.

The method of transmalleolar drilling has been discussed in Chapter VI. The use of the anterior arthroscopic cruciate ligament guide has helped considerably in developing this approach. The above techniques, as well as the passage of small instruments through transmalleolar channels, have been performed successfully on a few occasions and appear to be promising methods of gaining the best approach for accurate surgery, thus yielding better results (Figures 10-37 through 10-41).

The ability with arthroscopy to take a "second look" is a great advantage, and will allowing for future refinement of treatment. This has been illustrated on the single defect of the plafond (as noted in Chapter XI and in Figures 10-37 through 10-41).

Removal of loose chondral and osteochondral fragments is easier with these new methods, and is done arthroscopically with more assurance than by open procedures. The ability to view the posterior compartment with distraction of the joint from the anterior approach (or posterolateral portal), to view the anterior compartment from the posterior approach, and to retrieve loose bodies (Figures 10-31 through 10-36) adds further to treatment of these lesions. Also, one has confidence at the conclusion of the arthroscopic procedure that all of the loose bodies have indeed been removed.

Postoperative treatment should include early motion and weight bearing for most lesions, with exceptions. This would be best after the first two weeks. The need for immobilization and/or longterm nonweight bearing does not appear to be necessary. Parisien[24] has also arrived at this conclusion (independent of this author's opinion). The decreased trauma and reduced risks of arthroscopic surgery will also allow more aggressive rehabilitation.

The author has concluded from his experience that patients with reconstructed lesions (excision, debridement, abrasion, and drilling) should have immediate or early motion and begin weight bearing in approximately two weeks. This will allow enough time for the formation of a clot and organization of tissue in the defect. Participation in sports should be withheld appropriately, until the lesion is judged completely healed and the tissue is mature. Those patients with more extensive shallow lesions of the talus (over 1.5cm in diameter) should begin early motion, but maintain nonweight bearing following reconstruction and drilling for approximately eight to ten weeks. (case 6) Return to heavy work or any demanding activity should be slow, according to each individual case. Rehabilitation may require from several months to over one year.

Intact lesions in young patients that have been drilled should be casted for about eight to ten weeks, and then early motion and nonweight bearing should be employed, until healing is judged complete. Return to sports can best again be judged independently by clinical criteria, irrespective of the x-ray findings. It is best to wait until full rehabilitation of the extremity has occurred.

Bone scans are of no practical value in following progression of healing after surgery is done because the radiographic uptake remains pronounced.

Summary and Conclusions

1. Better evaluation of these lesions can be done arthroscopically with distraction.
2. Surgery is more accurate with the use of the distractor since there is more room to work and more accessibility from multiple portals.
3. The need for an osteotomy has been eliminated with these methods namely transmalleolar drilling and instrumentation.
4. There is more assurance of removal of associated loose bodies, especially in the posterior compartment with the combined use of the posterolateral and anterior approaches.
5. Earlier motion and weight bearing in most cases can be accomplished as a result of these methods.
6. "Second looks" are possible with arthroscopy allowing evaluation of the healing process.
7. Morbidity and the incidence of complications has been lessened considerably.

References

1. Alexander AH, Lichtman DM: Surgical Treatment of Transchondral Talar-Dome Fractures (Osteochondritis Dissecans). Am J Bone & Joint Surg 62-A:646-652, 1980.
2. Arcomano JP, Kamhi E, Karas S, et al.: Transchondral Fracture and Osteochondritis Dissecans of Talus. NY State J Med 78:2183-2189, 1978.
3. Berndt AL, Harty M: Transchondral Fractures (Osteochondritis Dissecans) of the Talus. Am J Bone & Joint Surg 41A:988-1017, 1959.
4. Barth A: Die Enstehung und das Wachsthum der frein Gelenkkor per. Arch. Klin. Chir., 56:507-573, 1898.
5. Blom JMH, Strijk SP: Lesions of the Trochlea Tali. Rad Clin 44:387-396, 1975.
6. Campbell CJ, Renawat CS: Osteochondritis Dissecans: The Question of Etiology. J Trauma 6 (2):201-21, 1966.
7. Canale ST, Belding RH: Osteochondral Lesions of the Talus. AM J Bone & Joint Surg 62-A:97-102, 1980.
8. Davidson AM, Steele HD, MacKenzie DA, et al.: A Review of Twenty-One Cases of Transchondral Fracture of the Talus. J Trauma 7:378-415, 1967.
9. Fisher AGJ: A study of loose bodies composed of cartilage or of cartilage and bone occurring in joints with special reference to their pathology and etiology. Brit. J. Surg 8:493-523, 1920-1921.
10. Goldsonte RA, Pisani AJ: Osteochondritis Dissecans of the Talus. NY State J Med 65:2487-2494, 1965.
11. Kappis M. Weiter beitrage sur traumatisch-mechanischen en tstehung der "spontanen" Knorpelablasungen (sogen, osteochondritis dissecans) Deutsche Zeitschr. Chir. 171:13-29, 1922 (Cited by Berndt and Harty [1]).
12. Konig F: Ueberfreie Korper in Den Gelenken. Dtsch Z Fuer chir 27:90, 1887-1888.

13. Lindholm TS, Osterman K, Vankka E: Osteochondritis Dissecans of Elbow, Ankle and Hip: A Comparison Survey. Clin Orth 148:245-253, 1980.
14. McCullough CJ, Venugopal V: Osteochondritis Dissecans of the Talus: The Natural History. Clin Orth 144:264-268, 1979.
15. Munro A, Alexander: Mocrigeologie, Berlin, Th. Billroth, 236, 1856. (Cited by Phemister [6]).
16. Naumetz VA, Schweigel JF: Osteocartilagenous Lesions of the Talar Dome. J Trauma 20:924-927, 1980.
17. O'Donoghue DH: Chondral and Osteochondral Fractures. J Trauma 6:469-481, 1966.
18. O'Farrell TA, Costello BG: Osteochondritis Dissecans of the Talus: The Late Results of Surgical Treatment. Br J Bone & Joint Surg 64-B:494-497, 1982.
19. Parisien S: Arthroscoppy of the Ankle: State of the Art. Con Orth 5:21-27, 1982.
20. Paul GR: Transchondral Fractures of the Talus. In: Ankle Injuries. Churchill Livingston, Inc. New York 113-130, 1983.
21. Rendu A: Fracture intra-articular parcellaire de la poulie astraglienne. Lyon Med., 150:220-222, 1932 (Cited by Berndt and Harty [2]).
22. Roden S, Tillegard P, Unander-Scharin L: Osteochondritis Dissecans and Similar Lesions of the Talus. Acta Orthop Scand. 23:51-66, 1953.
23. Scharling M: Osteochondritis Dissecans of the Talus. Acta Orthop Scand. 49:89-94, 1978.
24. Yao J, Weis E: Osteochondritis Dissecans. Orth Rev 14:190-204, 1985.
25. Yvars MF: Osteochondral Fractures of the Dome of the Talus. Clin Orth 114:185-191, 1976.
26. Phemister DB: The Causes of and Changes in Loose Bodies Arising from the Articular surfaces of the Joint. J Bone & Joint Surg. 6:278, 1924.

CHAPTER 11

OTHER CHONDRAL AND OSTEOCHONDRAL LESIONS

James F. Guhl, M.D.

This chapter will deal with lesions of chondral and osteochondral origin other than osteochondritis dissecans and osteochondral fractures of the talar dome. This will include chondral defects of the dome, chondral and osteochondral lesions of the plafond, osteophytes, loose bodies, degenerative or posttraumatic arthritis, fractures, postfracture defects and miscellaneous problems.

Chondral Lesions

Often the diagnosis of chondral pathology requires careful probing techniques. This method could not be employed as well until mechanical distraction and the use of the ankle holder had been developed. These innovations allowed the ankle to be held in a firm position with more space and ease of approach in which to work in the ankle joint. Initial debridement of synovial tissue and fibrocartilage may be necessary for adequate visualization. Evaluation of all chondral surfaces of the joint may then be accomplished. Careful observation is required to determine if the articular cartilage is soft, firm, loose, raised, depressed, or fibrillated. The use of methylane blue dye proved to be as helpful in the ankle as in the knee joint. A few ccs of concentrated methylene blue dye may be injected into the joint followed by irrigation and subsequent viewing. Another way is to instill a dilute solution for a few minutes and then flush it out of the joint. The application of light dimming techniques or tangential viewing with a 70 degree oblique arthroscope is also important.

Defects of the Talar Dome

Some defects of the talar dome may present for the first time arthroscopically. They should also be suspected in the presence of soft tissue pathology where they may coexist because of the mechanism of injury. Therefore their presence should be kept in mind when evaluating any form of the synovial impingement syndrome, adhesions, or chronic, nonspecific synovitis.

The surface area of the articular cartilage should be scrutinized for incongruities. The smallest amount of fibrous tissue protruding from any linear defect, the least movement or loosening, or loss of resiliency or luster should be suspected. Such areas can then be easily dissected with a probe from the surrounding normal healthy cartilage. More obvious stellate defects, linear cracks, and fibrillated necrotic areas may be seen. There are also clearcut distinct craters, with or without cartilagenous loose bodies. These appear to be more common in the talar dome than in the plafond. Most of these lesions require treatment.

X-ray evaluation begins with routine films, and, if negative, these should be followed by the usual positional views and special techniques described for osteochondritis dissecans. Stress films may help to predict the existence of these defects and their location by the areas of contact between the talus and plafond. Bone scans are negative, since there is only chondral involvement. Lateral arthrotomograms or contrast studies can often delineate these defects as well as identify chondral loose bodies. Beltram[1] describes a new technique, surface coil MR imagery, which may demonstrate pitting or destruction of the articular cartilage surface.

Some chondral lesions of the talar dome found initially at arthroscopy may actually be unrecognized small or shallow osteochondral fractures. In this case, the bone scan may be weakly positive due to limited bone involvement (or due to early minimal arthritic changes). For this reason both entities may not have been recognized on the original x-rays. Further factors added to this, regarding these defects, may have been inadequate x-ray techniques, lack of choice of the proper views, or failure to employ special procedures. In any event, these lesions are osteochondral fractures with a very small layer of bone on the undersurface. They may be intact, show signs of early separation, be partially detached, or free as "chondral" loose bodies.

Techniques of treatment require complete or adequate debridement of all necrotic or diseased articular cartilage, abrasion of the base, and drilling. Basket forceps and instruments developed for arthroscopic surgery of the ankle are necessary, as well as the small or large motorized instruments. Special instruments include various curettes, cartilage knives, and rasps. Drilling is done with an .062 Kirschner wire. Any combination of approaches that best suits the location may be used. The posterolateral portal is of value in studying lesions located in the posterior aspect of the dome. These posterior defects are usually medial in location, but lateral lesions have been encountered, including cysts of the talus that may require drilling alone. The transmalleolar approaches (described in Chapter VI) may be necessary to gain access and to obtain the best possible angle of approach for surgery. The articular cartilage overlying these cysts is usually intact. The cysts may be drilled by reference from the x-ray views, utilizing the arthroscopic anterior cruciate ligament guide for placement of the Kirschner wire. Of course, larger cysts will require open bone grafting.

Lesions of the Plafond

Chondral defects of the plafond are probably the most difficult lesions to diagnose in the ankle joint. They cannot be detected by any x-ray views and the bone scan is negative since there is only chondral involvement. Theoretically, the arthrotomogram or contrast studies should delineate these defects, but often these studies have not proven to be of practical application. Here again, surface coil MR imagery may be helpful, as recently shown. Until distraction, arthroscopic detection has been limited. Nevertheless, these lesions do occur as a result of impaction, compression, or twisting injuries. Here the talus is driven up or impacted against the plafond. They may occur in the presence of more extensive fractures of the extremity and be overlooked or not considered at the time of the injury. The defects can be the source of chondral loose bodies, and they can also set the stage for arthritic changes in the ankle joint in future years.

Suspicion of the existence of these chondral lesions may be one of the best indications for arthroscopy of the ankle. They may appear as large stellate lesions or irregular defects with surrounding areas of loose necrotic cartilage. At other times a clearcut defect with or without a separated or loose body (bodies) is noted. On occasion, areas of chondromalacia and fibrillation may present, making the diagnosis more difficult. After the chondromalacia is debrided, the defect then becomes apparent from the surrounding normal articular cartilage.

Large osteochondral lesions may also occur. These defects of the plafond may be discovered and distinguished from lesions of the talar dome by the bone scan. Better localization is obtained by the utilization of pin hole collimation or SPECT (photon emission computer tomography), when these lesions are not visible on routine x-ray views. Further confirmation is done by the use of tomography, CT scan, or, again, surface coil MR imagery.

Treatment requires complete debridement, abrasion, and drilling. The defect should be trimmed back to healthy articular cartilage with a perpendicular margin. Drilling is recommended because of the author's past experience in defects of the talus and other joint surfaces. The open drilling technique has been recommended for osteochondritis dissecans and other such lesions for years, as shown by a review of the literature. It is also more logical from a scientific standpoint. According to Cheung,[2] more Type II fibrocartilage is found, consisting of a greater percentage of hyaline material, when this method is utilized experimentally. These lesions can be approached for surgery and drilled from the anterior portals with distraction. The posterior approaches are not necessary and are of no use because of the anatomical configuration of the talocrural joint.

Postoperative rehabilitation requires early active motion, plus stretching and strengthening exercises. A period of approximately eight to ten weeks of nonweight bearing is more important here, as compared to defects of the dome (except in large shallow lesions of that structure). CPM (continued passive motion) may be considered in the future as these treatment methods are further developed.

There has been only one case in the author's experience where a "second look" was done five months after surgery. The articular surface of the plafond improved, but the fibrocartilage appeared to be only fair in quality. More time may have been required for this tissue to mature. Other cases treated in the same fashion had good clinical results at longterm followup, up to two years later.

While little knowledge about this pathology is known, it must be assumed that nature probably took care of some of these lesions in the past, at least to some degree. Also, it has been known that the ankle joint has been quite "forgiving" regarding arthritic changes. However, serious considerations should now be given regarding treatment when this type of pathology is encountered in a symptomatic ankle or in conjunction with other lesions.

Loose Bodies

The origin, development, and fate of loose bodies should be kept in mind when reviewing the history, physical findings, and planning treatment according to Milgram.[3] Loose bodies originate from chondral and osteochondral defects (osteochondritis dissecans and osteochondral fractures), osteophytes, degenerative arthritis, and synovial chondromatosis. They may enlarge by osteoblastic formation or decrease in size by osteoclastic activity. They may become attached to the synovium and later revascularize, be absorbed, or possibly break loose again. Damage to the articular cartilage can be minimal in some cases and more extensive in others. Loose bodies appear to be found with equal incidence in the anterior and posterior compartment of the ankle joint with minimal room to lodge elsewhere. In these locations, they can be hidden by numerous synovial folds or adhesions.

In addition to routine x-rays and positional views, contrast arthrography is helpful. Cineradiography may be considered, but has limited value in the author's experience.

In general, loose body removal is much preferred by the arthroscopic method rather than by arthrotomy. In addition to other disadvantages, the latter will give no more assurance of complete removal if one or a number of these lesions are encountered. Complete arthroscopic search for a single or remaining loose body will afford a much greater promise of success, since the development of the distraction method. Mechanical distraction, with full distention, employment of the ankle holder, utilization of all available approaches, and the ability to triangulate in the posterior compartment as well as the anterior space will aid considerably in mobilization and successful removal of these lesions.

The portals used most are the anterolateral and anteromedial. At times, the anterocentral and posterolateral portals are of help, particularly if the loose body is lodged posterior. These latter two approaches are also best for the passage of instruments. Even the posteromedial portal can be utilized for manipulating a probe or small instrument, if one is careful, skillful, and the occasion demands. A good example of this would be the need to recover a small fragment from a broken instrument in this location. If a particular approach has limitations, there are other choices. Triangulation can be accomplished by many different combinations.

It is elementary but important to remember to immediately turn off the inflow and outflow and completely distend the ankle, if one is having problems. In difficult cases, air or gas arthroscopy may be worth considering. Small chondral loose bodies can be removed from the joint by suction or with the motorized shaver.

Osteophytes

Anterior Impingement Lesions

Osteophytes of the ankle are amenable to arthroscopic treatment as was first suspected. Bartlett[4] described their occurrence as the "anterior impingement syndrome." This is a condition that occurs with extreme dorsiflexion of the ankle and results in formation of the impingement osteophyte. It is one cause of repeated ankle pain and various degrees of limitation of motion. The condition is commonly seen in athletes. O'Donoghue[5] reported a 45% incidence in football players, and Stoller et al.[6] reported 59.3% in dancers. These spurs form as the result of direct trauma following forced dorsiflexion of the foot, according to O'Donoghue[5] or as the result of capsular traction following extensive plantar flexion. Marginal osteophytes seem to occur as the result of the healing process. Also, with repeated trauma these exostoses can form along the anterior margin of the medial malleolus or fibula.

Previously, an open incision was indicated after failure of conservative treatment such as injections, antiinflammatory medications, physical therapy, and various forms of immobilization and padding. Arthroscopic surgical techniques are now applicable instead of open treatment in a number of cases. Open treatment requiring extensive dissection can be done, if the above fails or does not seem initially indicated.

According to Bartlett,[4] clinical complaints in this syndrome are "pain in dorsiflexion resulting in difficulty with: stair climbing, walking up hills, squatting and sprinting". The pain is worse with activity and may be noted as recurrent ankle sprains. There is often a long delay in diagnosing these conditions. The diagnosis is made, according to Bartlett,[4] by: "pain with passive dorsiflexion, tenderness to palpation along the anterior tibial tendon of the joint, a loss of motion, and radiological evidence of impingement with an exostosis or "loose body". The author of this text recommends lateral flexion extension views for preoperative evaluation and postoperative followup. The bone scan is also helpful in indicating the presence of osteophytes. Pin hole collimation or SPECT will help in better localization, as well as the CT scan and MRI.

Arthroscopic treatment is carried out with the extremity placed in the ankle holder and the joint distracted. Excision of this lesion could be accomplished without the above, but its utilization allows for more expeditious surgery, less scuffing, and a complete evaluation of the joint and subsequent treatment. The three anterior portals are used, along with the posterolateral portal, for further exploration, as necessary. Often, there are other interarticular lesions that have to be treated. The joint must often be initially debrided by performing a synovectomy of the anterior compartment. Excision is aided by some limited stripping of the capsule, as necessary. The use of the downbiting rongeur, osteotome, rasps, and curettes, as well as the small or large joint power system, is required. Postoperative management includes a soft compression dressing, early active range of motion and strengthening exercises with weight bearing, as indicated. In advance cases, arthrotomy may be required with both anterolateral and anteromedial incisions, as necessary. The osteophyte may be excised from both approaches. Motion should be checked during surgery to see if extension has been regained.

Early results of Bartlett's[4] series are encouraging (as well as the author's experience) in that most patients had responded or improved in their symptoms and about half showed increased motion in dorsiflexion. The rate of recurrence and longterm results is unknown. It may be that arthroscopic treatment, being less traumatic, with less morbidity and an earlier return to normal function, will result in a shorter course of rehabilitation and, perhaps, a lower recurrence rate.

Posterior Impingement Lesions

There are certain osteochondral impingement lesions of the posterior compartment of which one should be aware. These are in addition to the soft tissue impingement entities mentioned in Chapter IX as amenable to arthroscopic intervention. Schonholtz[7] mentioned "osteophyte" of the posterior lip. Hamilton[8] referred to a large posteromedial lip present on the back of the talus causing a posterior medial impingement (See Chapter VIII). These structures are interarticular in location. Symptomatic nonunions of the posterior facet (attachment of the posterior talofibular ligament) can occur. Posterior lateral lesions, such as those involving the os trigonum or trigonal process (Steida's process), are extraarticular and may cause symptoms in the hind foot according to Parks.[9] If not well seen on routine x-rays, they can be discovered by the bone scan and better demonstrated by CT scan or MRI. Treatment of these pathological lesions is done by open intervention through arthroscopy may be of further aide in diagnosis.

Traumatic and Degenerative Arthritis

Arthroscopic treatment of the arthritic ankle was initially considered worthless by this author. Experience with arthritic knees generated much initial enthusiasm, some over-treatment, and later disappointment. It than became evident that, with proper selection, some indications could be developed. Cases of arthritis of the ankle that should be excluded from arthroscopic intervention are those with advanced destruction, marked joint line narrowing, extensive fibrosis, and a significant degree of instability or deformity. Patients presenting with ankles having some limited motion due to capsulitis, a minimal to moderate degree of fibroarthrosis, osteophytes, chondral defects, loose bodies and only a minimal degree of instability, would be candidates for arthroscopic surgery. Also, to be considered when contemplating arthroscopic treatment of degenerative arthritis of the ankle, are the degree of disability, alternative forms of treatment, results of previous treatment, type of job demand, and expected result. Finally, a cooperative patient with a positive attitude and reasonable expectations should be considered a candidate for this type of surgery.

At times results may be very favorable and at other times there may only be a limited degree of improvement. Partial recovery may be much appreciated and allow continued function and employment. The result may be further enhanced with the aid of antiinflammatory medications, aspirin, or other means to keep these patients comfortable. Overtreatment for this condition should be carefully avoided. It should also be remembered that the x-ray picture of arthritis of the ankle does not always correlate with the symptoms. Some patients with advanced x-ray findings and longstanding involvement may often be relatively asymptomatic.

In selecting cases of ankle arthritis, the above indications and conditions should be kept in mind. The symptoms should be longstanding and the disability significant. Then, failure to respond to conservative treatment is considered a prime indication. Expected results should always be clearly outlined to the patient.

The pathological components of the arthritic ankle, as viewed from the arthroscopic standpoint, should be considered separately for treatment and the total picture assessed. These are defects of any surface, as described. Included are chondromalacia, osteophytes, loose bodies, chondral and osteochondral defects. Treatment of all of the above has been individually discussed previously. Of additional consideration is extensive chronic synovitis, the synovial impingement lesion (local or general), adhesions, fibroarthrosis, and, in some cases, capsulitis. Extensive debridement with motorized equipment and lavage is required. The distraction method has further contributed to the treatment of capsulitis with limited motion. This is done along with manipulation and excision of osteophytes.

Finally the use of careful remodeling of the articular cartilage with small joint instruments (rasps, burrs, arthroscopic osteotomes, baskets, and knives) is important. Areas of degenerative cartilage will require more extensive debridement, abrasion, and drilling, in some cases. The postoperative use of interarticular steroids in selected cases where there is existing articular damage and extensive synovial involvement should be considered. On occasion, installation of 0.5% Marcaine with 1 to 200,000 epinephrine and a steroid into the joint may be helpful to reduce postoperative bleeding and further adhesion formation. Early mobility may then be regained. Immediate postoperative use of ice packs and early motion, plus heat modalities later for rehabilitation, are suggested. Progressive range of motion, strengthening, and stretching exercises in a progressive manner should be performed daily. The continuous passive motion machine for the ankle may be advisable in the future for selected cases, when a more extensive abrasion is performed.

Fractures, Postfracture Pathology, and Miscellaneous Conditions

In addition to interarticular lesions of the talus and plafond, there are other sequelae of fracture trauma that may become chronically symptomatic. These are: a medial or lateral talomalleolar diastasis; an oblique fracture of the fibula, extending into the lateral corner of the ankle joint and causing the formation of an interarticular osteochondral and soft tissue impingement; a postsurgical or posttraumatic synostosis, extending into the joint (and others). Arthroscopic debridement of the capsular, ligamentous, and synovial material and osteocartilagenous tissue or debris from these painful areas often will bring relief.

Ferkel[10] demonstrated the utilization of arthroscopic techniques in treating acute fractures extending into the ankle joint, just as others have done regarding fractures (of the tibial plateau) of the knee joint. The need for its practical application will be shown by future experience.

Case Reviews

Lesions of the Talar Dome

Case 1 J.K. For clinical history please see Figures 11-1 and 11-2.

Case 2 C.D. For clinical history please see Figure 11-3.

Lesions of the Tibial Plafond

Case 3 L.P. (Figures 11-4 and 11-5). This 47-year-old laborer has been treated for an undisplaced hairline fracture of the distal fibula. The extremity was placed in a plaster cast for the appropriate period of time. After rehabilitation, he still had pain in the posterior lateral aspect of the ankle joint that persisted for several months. He was unable to work. Repeat x-rays showed complete healing of the fracture. The examination was not remarkable, except for tenderness in the lateral aspect of the ankle. Pain in that area was particularly aggravated by motion in all planes. An arthroscopic examination was performed, and, immediately upon distracting the joint, a large chondral fragment was noted in a defect in the posterolateral corner of the tibial plafond. This was removed arthroscopicaly with a grasping forceps, utilizing the anterolateral and anteromedial portals. The arthroscope and instruments were alternated between the two approaches, and the base of the crater was debrided, abraded, and drilled. The joint was then thoroughly irrigated. The patient was placed in a compression dressing for five days and was on crutches for about two weeks. He returned to normal activity and on followup one year later had only minimal aching. He was improved to a satisfactory degree with arthroscopic treatment.

Loose Bodies

Case 4 A.B. For clinical history please see Figure 11-6.

Case 5 F.R. (Figures 11-7 through 11-10). The patient was referred to this author with recurrent pain and locking of the left ankle joint. This existed for years and became disabling. Clinical examination was not remarkable, but x-rays showed a large loose body in the posterior aspect of the joint. Arthroscopy was performed with distraction, the use of the ankle holder, and utilization of the posterolateral approach, as well as the anterocentral portal. Evaluation of the ankle joint was not remarkable, except for a minimal reactive synovitis and a large loose body located posteriorly. With the aid of maximum distraction, the fragment could be grasped in the posterior compartment, but not pulled through the joint and out through the anterocentral approach. The loose body was then viewed via the arthroscope through the central approach. A grasping forceps was placed in the posterolateral portal. The fragment was then teased into the jaws of the forceps by a hypodermic needle inserted anteriorly, and it was pulled out through the posterolateral aspect of the ankle. Another small chondral loose body was flushed out of the joint. To date the patient has done well.

Case 6 T.T. For clinical history please see Figures 11-11 and 11-12.

Case 7 M.N. For clinical history please see Figures 11-13 through 11-21.

Osteophytes

Case 8 N.L. (Figures 11-22 through 11-27). This 28-year-old man was referred to the author with a history of stabbing pain in the anterior aspect of the left ankle. This was of particular concern to him since he was a kicker on a professional football team. He had been to several sports medicine centers around the country and received conservative treatment with no improvement. His performance was gradually deteriorating regarding his distance and "hang time." The pain in the "plant" foot disrupted his timing in that when he would get into position to kick, the pain would shoot up his leg and distract his concentration. Clinical evaluation showed anterior tenderness and pain in that area on manipulation of the foot. This was aggravated by dorsiflexion. X-rays showed a minimal degree of degenerative changes of the tibiotalar joint, as well as a large anterior osteophyte. At arthroscopy the osteophyte was removed with a rongeur and modeled with a rasp and the use of the small joint power instruments. The patient was discharged wearing a compression dressing, with directions to use a crutch when walking and avoid weightbearing. He developed some drainage due to overactivity early in the postoperative period. Cultures were negative and the symptoms rapidly improved. The following season the patient led his conference in kicking and was selected for the all pro team.

Case 9 R.B. For clinical history please see Figures 11-28 and 11-29.

Case 10 J.W. For clinical history please see Figures 11-30 and 11-31.

Degenerative Arthritis

Case 11 P.P. (Figures 11-32 through 11-38). This 48-year-old man was referred by another orthopedic surgeon. He originally sustained a fracture at the lower right tibia and multiple other fractures in an industrial injury. He continued to have pain in the right ankle joint. Examination showed that the ankle was almost completely devoid of motion, except for a few remaining degrees. There was pain on manipulation and local anterior tenderness. The patient also walked with a distinct limp. X-rays showed some narrowing of the ankle joint with a large anterior osteophyte, as well as a spur of the neck of the talus and further degenerative changes. It was the author's initial opinion that the patient would not be a good candidate for arthroscopic surgery. Further conservative treatment brought no improvement, and the patient then was finally arthroscoped with distraction.

Examination showed marked chondromalacia of the lateral aspect of the joint, comprising approximately 30% of the tibial plafond. There were minimal changes scattered in the dome of the talus. The ankle was distracted, and the area of the plafond was debrided with a shaver and trimmer. It then became apparent that the area of fibrillated cartilage was in fact a large chondral defect of the articular cartilage of the lower tibia. After continued exploration with the probe, debridement with the power instruments, and, finally, the curette and basket forceps, a well defined defect was exposed. The remaining surrounding articular cartilage was sharply demarcated and in fairly good condition. Further debridement was done to clear the joint of associated reactive synovitis. The base of the cortical defect was abraded and drilled. Arthroscopic excision of the anterior osteophyte was done. The joint was then manipulated.

Following surgery, the patient had some decrease in pain and a significant increase in his ankle motion, except for the last few degrees of extension. He required another surgical procedure at a later date at which time he had open excision of the remaining portion of the osteophyte (Figure 11-38). At that time a repeat arthroscopic examination of the right ankle was performed. This showed fair fibrocartilage in the defect of the tibial plafond. If a few more months had elapsed, perhaps the cartilage would have matured further.

It appears that certain cases of degenerative arthritis of the ankle will be amenable to arthroscopic surgery, particularly if this is considered separately for a combination of defects, as mentioned above. If there is advanced degeneration of the joint, advanced fibrosis, deformity or instability, the indications for arthroscopic intervention would be more doubtful. A limited abrasion arthroplasty might be of some help, as shown in a small number of cases by the author and others. Further experience is necessary to substantiate the value of this type of treatment.

Fractures, Post-fractures, Pathology, and Miscellaneous Conditions

Case 12 M.R. For clinical history please see Figures 11-39 through 11-45.

Case 13 T.F. For clinical history please see Figures 11-46 through 11-49.

Case 14 P.L. For clinical history please see Figure 11-50.

Case 15 R.W. For clinical history please see Figure 11-51.

Case 16 J.B. For clinical history please see Figure 11-52.

References
1. Beltran J, Notor AM, Mosure JC, et al. Ankle: Surface Coil MR Imaging At 1.5Tl. Rad 161:203-209, 1986.
2. Cheung HS, Cottrell WH, Stephenson K, et al.: In Vitro Collagen Biosynthesis In Healing And Normal Rabbit Articular Cartilage. J Bone & Joint Surg 60A(8):1076-1081, 1978.
3. Milgram JW: The Classification of Loose Bodies in Human Joints. Clin Orth 124:282-291, 1977.
4. Bartlett, R. AAOS Exhibit, New Orleans, February 1986.
5. O'Donoghue DH: Chondral and Osteochondral Fractures. J Trauma 6:469-481, 1966.
6. Stoller SM: A Comparative Study of the Frequency of Anterior Impingement Exostosis of the Ankle in Dancer and Non Dancer Foot and Ankle. Vol. 4, p. 201-203, 1984.
7. Schonholtz G.J: Arthroscopic Surgery of the Shoulder, Elbow and Ankle. Springfield, IL, Charles C. Thomas, 1986.
8. Hamilton: Personal Communication, 1986.
9. Parks JC: Injuries of the Hindfoot. Clin Orth 122:28-36, January 1977.
10. Ferkel R: Personal Communication, 1987.

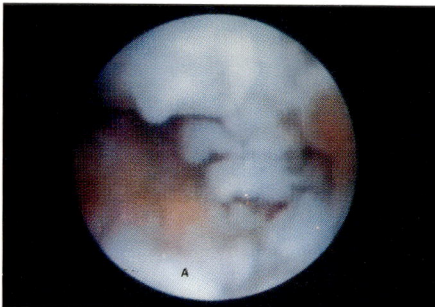

Figure 9-1. Arthroscopic view of a case of rheumatoid synovitis (and arthritis) of the right ankle. Note the villi formation. A, talus. (Courtesy of J.S. Parisien.)

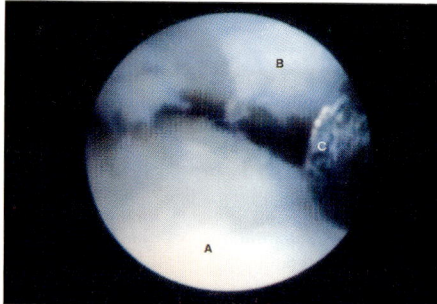

Figure 9-2. Arthroscopic view of the same case. The involvement of the articular cartilage of the dome of the talus (A) is clearly shown. B, anterior tibia; C, cannula. (Courtesy of J.S. Parisien.)

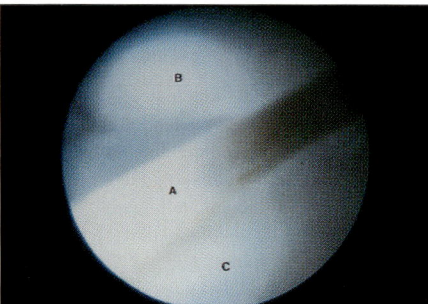

Figure 9-3. This adhesion (A) is located in the anterior aspect of the right ankle. It occurred in a young man who complained of severe intermittent pain associated with locking. The adhesion was removed arthroscopically and the patient was cured. There were no other lesions recognized. B, anterior tibia; C, talus.

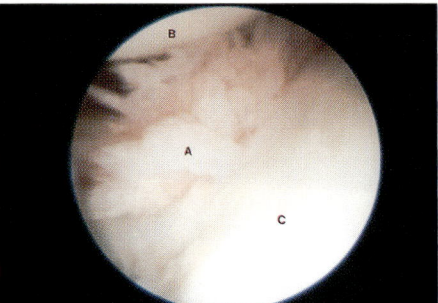

Figure 9-4. This example of a local subacute synovitis (A) is typical of what occurs a few months following a sprain of the right ankle. At a later date it may become chronic and develop into a synovial impingement lesion. B, fibula; C, talus.

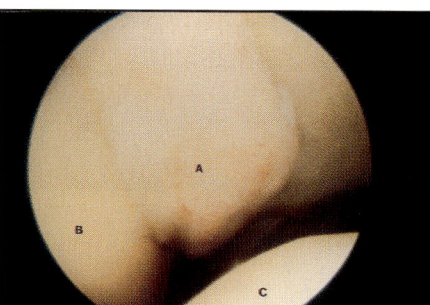

Figure 9-5. An example of a typical synovial impingement lesion of the right ankle. Note the hemorrhage and pigmentation on the surface. It is attached to the superior portion of the plafond at its lateral aspect adjacent to the fibula. This appears to develop from the synovial recess in the superior portion of the lateral talomalleolar joint. A, soft tissue impingement; B, fibula; C, talus.

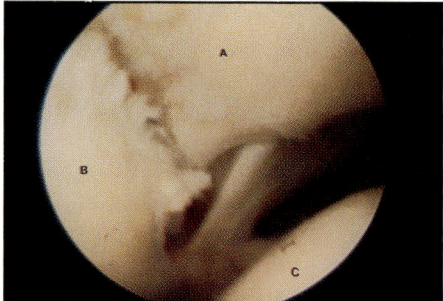

Figure 9-6. This postoperative view shows complete excision of this soft tissue mass. A, plafond; B, fibula; C, talus.

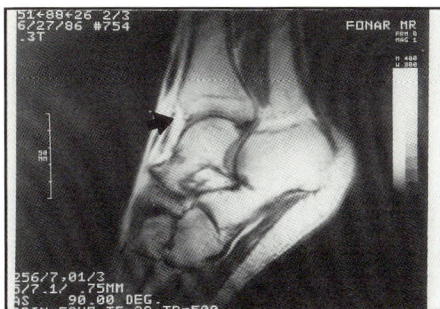

Figure 9-7. This arrow shows the anterior capsular syndrome (soft tissue impingement syndrome) as seen with MRI. (Courtesy of B.R. Mandelbaum.)

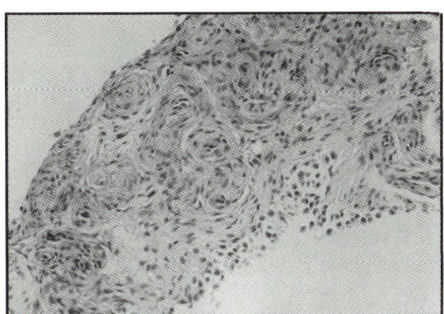

Figure 9-8. This is an example of prominent subsynovial blood vessel proliferation (IOOX;H^E). (Courtesy of R. Ferkel and D. Kasamain.)

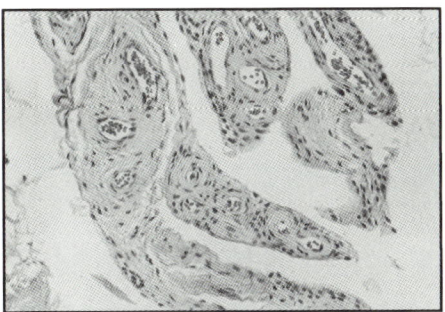

Figure 9-9. Papillary change (hyperplasia) of synovium (IOOX; H^E). (Courtesy of R. Ferkel and D. Kasamain.)

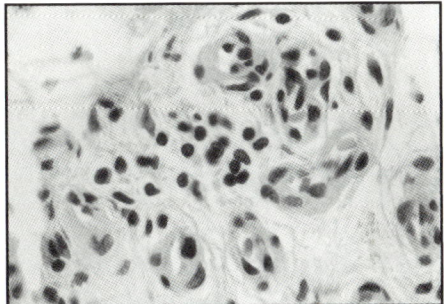

Figure 9-10. Chronic inflammation was minimal, consisting primarily of a few lymphocytes (200X; H^E). (Courtesy of R. Ferkel and D. Kasamain.)

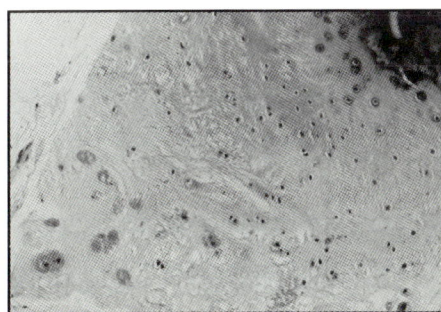

Figure 9-11. Hyaline cartilage demonstrating degenerative change (IOOX;H & E). (Courtesy of R. Ferkel and D. Kasamain.)

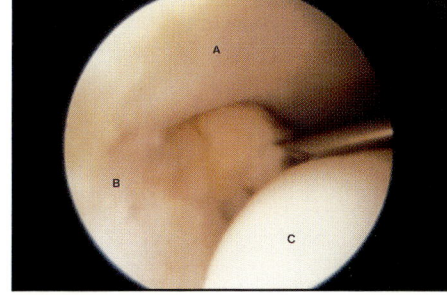

Figure 9-12. This is an example of a typical soft tissue impingement lesion located in the posterolateral corner of the right ankle. The patient had longstanding localized pain and tenderness. Complete relief was obtained after excision. A, plafond; B, fibula; C, talus.

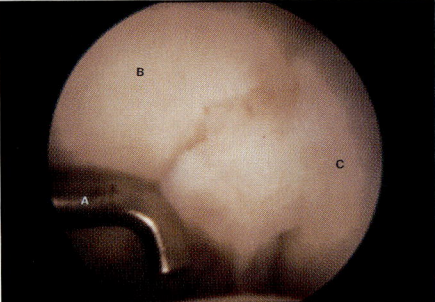

Figure 9-13. Posterolateral synovial impingement lesion (left ankle). The probe (A) is valuable in determining the extent of the lesion. B, plafond; C, fibula; D, talus.

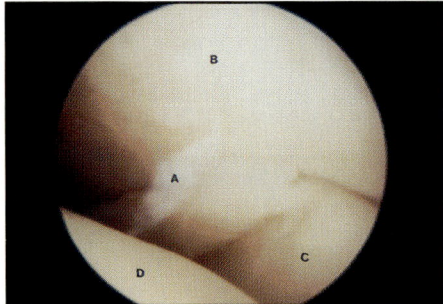

Figure 9-14. This is another example of a posterolateral soft tissue lesion (A) of the left ankle joint. B, plafond; C, fibula; D, talus.

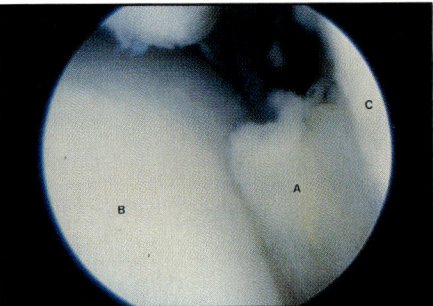

Figure 9-15. A meniscoid (A) of the left ankle in a young woman. Removal gave significant relief. B, talus; C, medial malleolus.

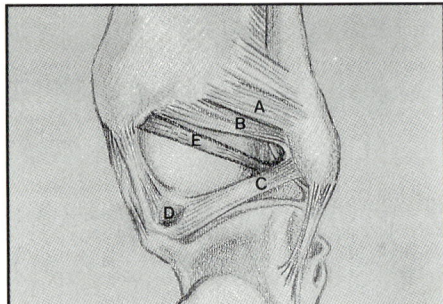

Figure 9-16. This diagram shows the location of a posterior tibiofibular ligament (A), a transverse tibiofibular ligament (B) as seen in the posterior compartment (as in Figure 3-18), a view of the tibial slip (E), the posterior talofibular ligament (C), and the os tirgonum (D).

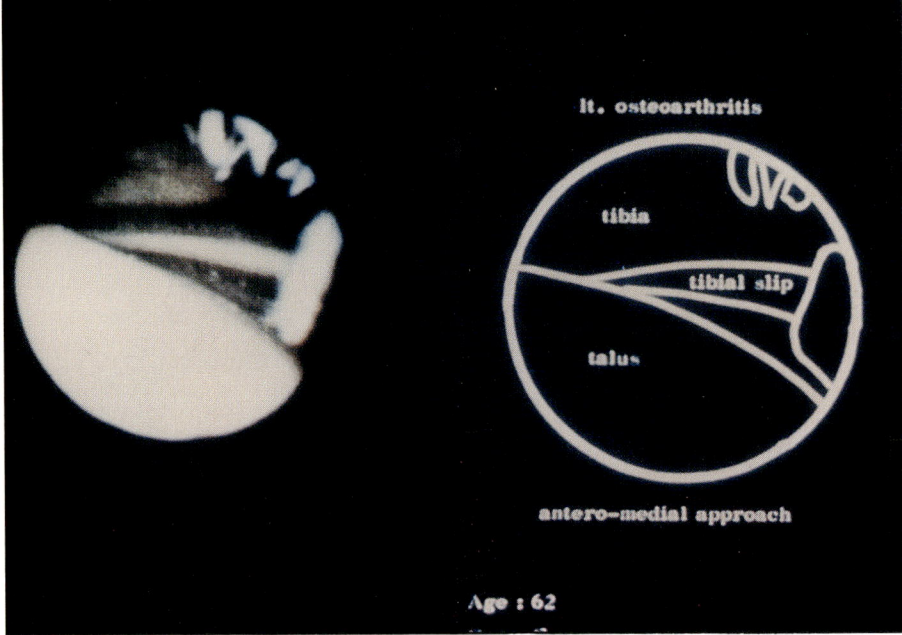

Figure 9-17. One of Dr.Ikeuchi's illustrations showing the "tibial slip". The structure is an extension of the transverse tibiofibular ligament.

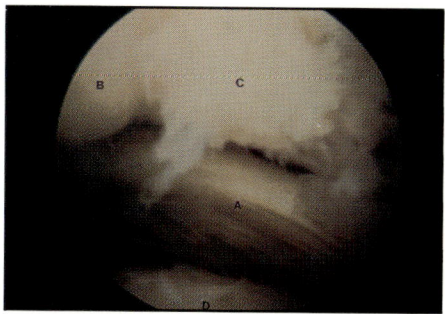

Figure 9-18. An example of an enlarged transverse tibiofibular ligament (A) in the posterior compartment of the left ankle joint as seen arthroscopically. It may be considered pathological when other lesions are ruled out and the symptoms are directly related to this structure. Excision should then be considered. B, plafond; C, synovitis; D, talus.

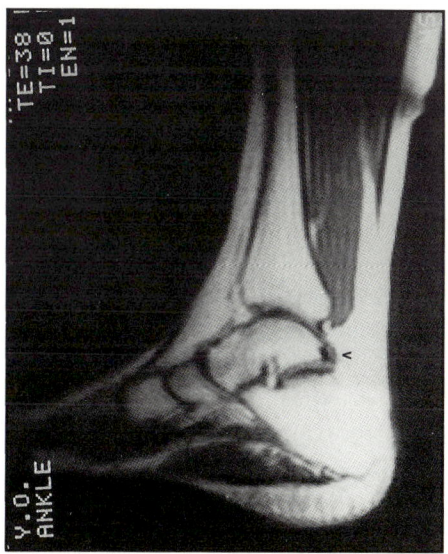

Figure 9-19. MRI. The arrow shows the location of the meniscus. (Courtesy of M. Meyerson.)

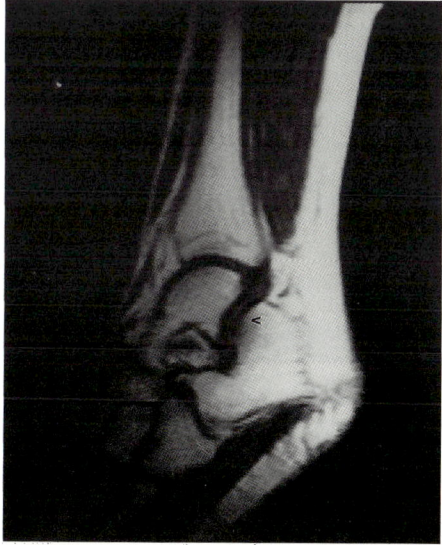

Figure 9-20. MRI. The arrow shows the location of the meniscus. (Courtesy of M. Meyerson.)

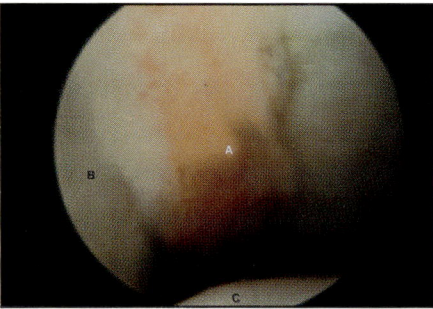

Figure 9-21. A typical synovial impingement lesion of the lateral aspect of the right ankle. It arises from the synovial recess of the superior portion of the lateral talomalleolar joint and extends from the anterior to the posterior aspect of the joint. Note the hemosiderin pigment. A, soft tissue impingement; B, fibula; C, talus.

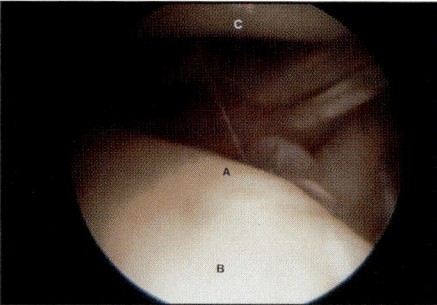

Figure 9-22. Arthroscopic view of the same ankle showing the medial surface of the talus. There was a loose fragment of articular cartilage noted. This chondral fracture (A) occurred when the talus (B) was tilted laterally at the time of injury and struck the tibial plafond (C), above.

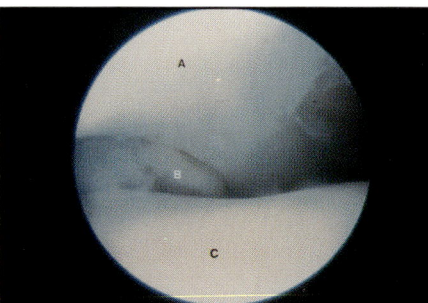

Figure 9-23. A case of a soft tissue impingement lesion in the posterolateral aspect of the right ankle joint. It is typical of this pathological entity. The patient had disabling pain completely relieved with excision. A, plafond; B, ganglion; C, talus.

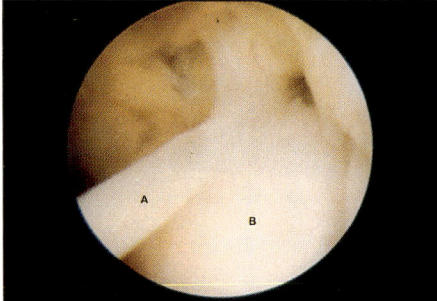

Figure 9-24. This adhesion (A) was found and shown arthroscopically in the anterior aspect of the left ankle joint of a 34-year-old woman. It caused pain, locking, buckling, and a feeling of instability. B, anterior talar dome.

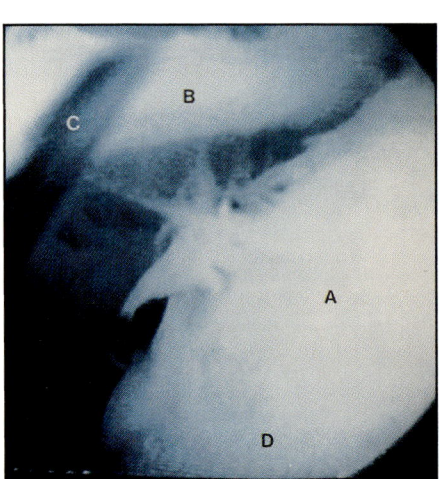

Figure 9-25. This view shows a chondral defect (A) caused by local trauma of the adjacent adhesion (B), which is lifted away from the cartilage surface by a hypodermic needle (C). On further exploration of the joint, seven other large adhesions were found. Clicking persisted until all adhesions were removed. The patient, whose condition improved considerably, remains satisfied two years after the operation. D, anterior talar dome.

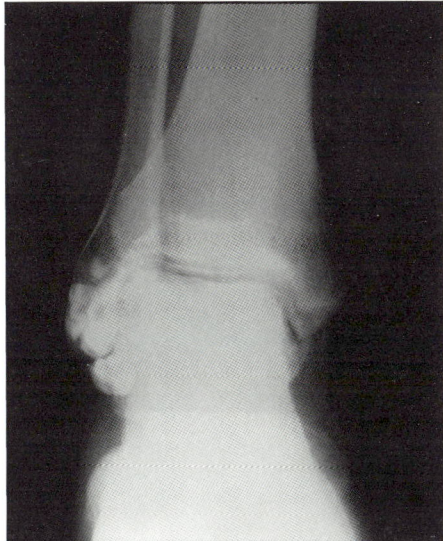

Figure 9-26. An AP arthrogram showing an example of synovial chondromatosis in the posterolateral aspect of the right ankle. This was not seen on routine x-ray views.

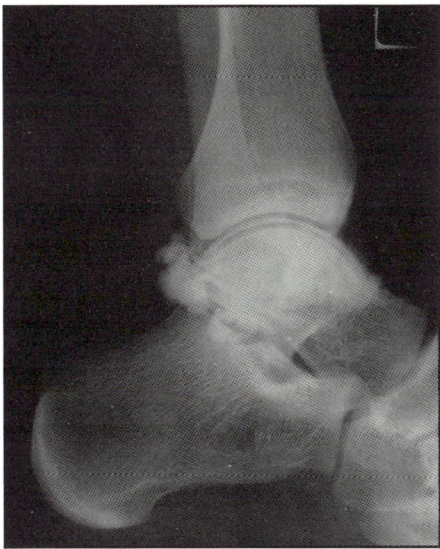

Figure 9-27. This lateral arthrogram shows the synovial chondromatosis, again in the posterolateral corner.

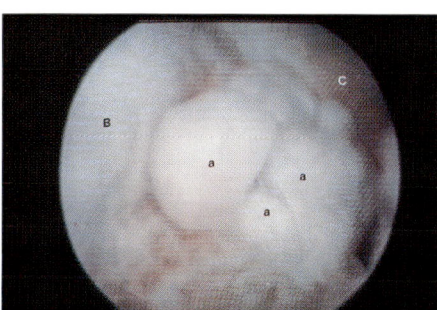

Figure 9-28. An arthroscopic view with several small loose bodies (A) located in the anterior ankle joint. B, anterior talar dome; C, anterior capsule.

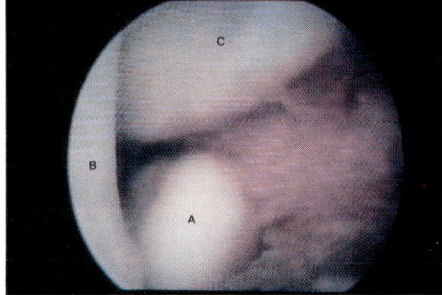

Figure 9-29. A view of the same case with a loose body (A) in the medial talomalleolar joint. B, talus; C, medial malleolus.

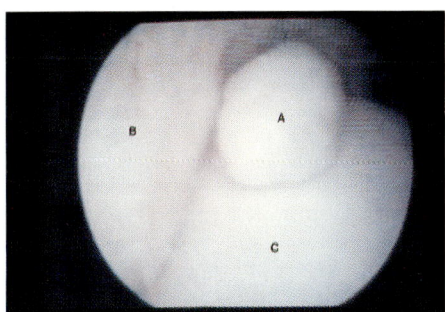

Figure 9-30. Another view showing a loose body (A) in the anterior recess in front of the tibia (B). Removal of all loose bodies, especially those posterior, was possible with mechanical distraction. C, anterior talar dome.

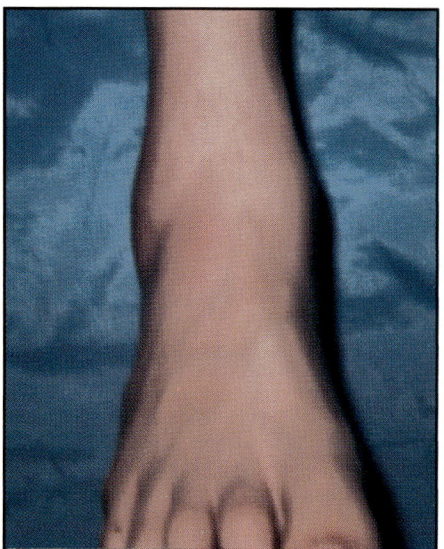

Figure 9-31. This is the right ankle of a 15-year-old boy who sustained a football injury six months prior to being examined by the author. He had intermittent and increasing pain. The patient finally presented with an acute septic ankle most likely hematogenous in origin. The bone scan showed a marked uptake.

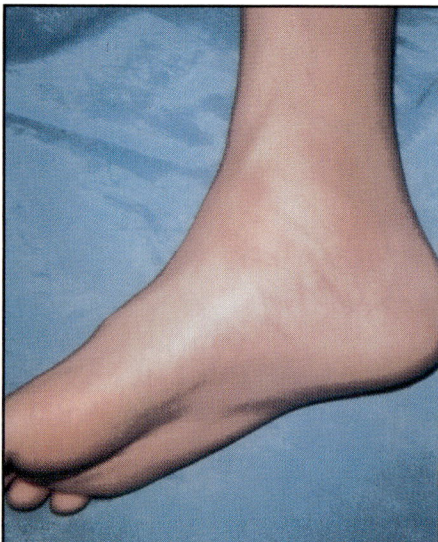

Figure 9-32. Another view of the same ankle.

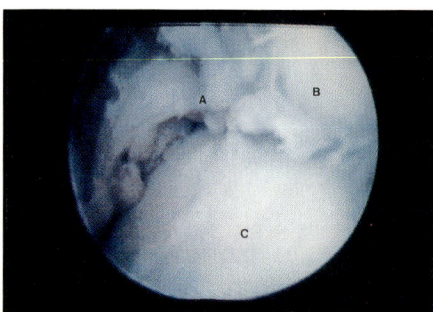

Figure 9-33. An arthroscopic view. Note the soft tissue (A) involvement, with little articular damage. B, anterior tibia; C, anterior talar dome.

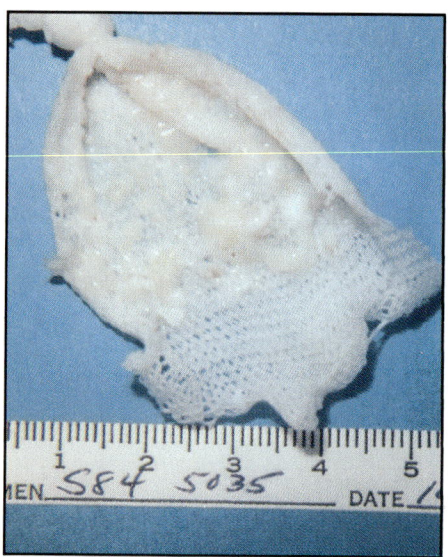

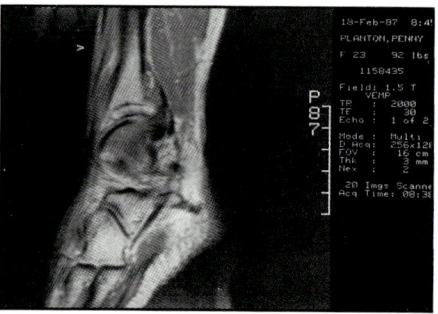

Figure 9-34. This specimen is shown in the gauze bag where it was collected from the suction tube at surgery. A complete debridement of the inflamed and infected synovial tissue was performed arthroscopically. The patient improved rapidly. He was in the hospital for one week with intravenous antibiotics and then discharged. He remained improved two years later.

Figure 9-35. MRI. This arrow shows tendinitis of the common extensor tendon.

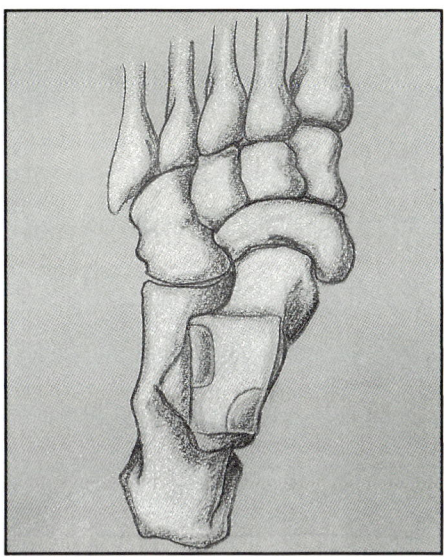

Figure 10-1. This diagram, modified by Paul,[20] shows the location of osteochondritis dissecans in the medial and lateral aspects of the talar dome.

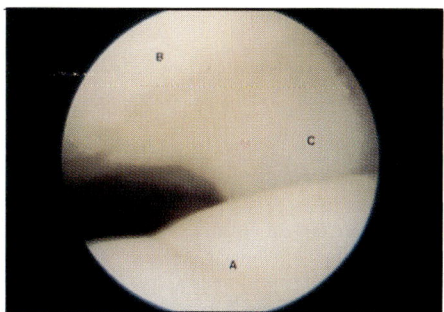

Figure 10-2. This is an arthroscopic view of an intact lesion in a young patient. There is slight bulging or elevation of the lesion, which is magnified to some degree by the arthroscope. However, the entire border was intact, and there was no break in the articular cartilage. The lesion was firm in its bed when probed. Transmalleolar drilling in situ is the treatment of choice, especially in young patients with large lesions. A, intact osteochondritis lesion; B, plafond; C, medial malleolus.

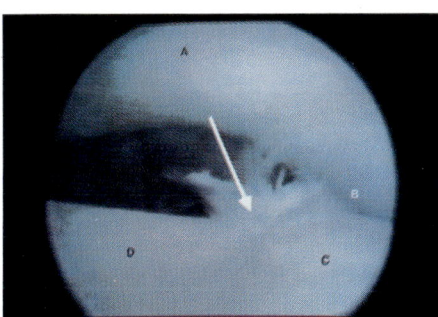

Figure 10-3. This is a video arthroscopic view of osteochondritis dissecans of the medial dome of the talus, showing partial separation. Note the break in the articular cartilage at the border of the lesion, which shows fibrous tissue protruding. When probed, this lesion appears to be slightly loose, indicating early separation. The treatment in this case is complete excision, debridement, abrasion, and drilling of the base. Arrow, fibrous margin; A, plafond; B, medial malleolus; C, separated osteochondritis lesion; D, dome of talus.

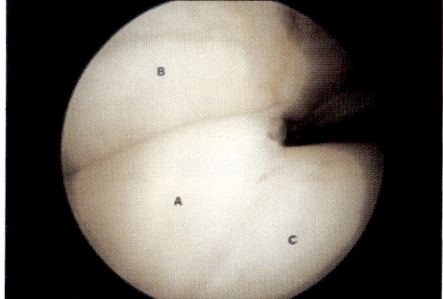

Figure 10-4. This is an arthroscopic view of a separated osteochondritis lesion (A). The break in the cartilage is complete. The fragment was easily lifted from its bed with a probe. Again, reconstruction (excision, debridement, abrasion and drilling) of the defect is the treatment of choice. Postoperatively, early motion and weight bearing was employed at about two weeks, with a good result. B, medial malleolus, C, dome of talus.

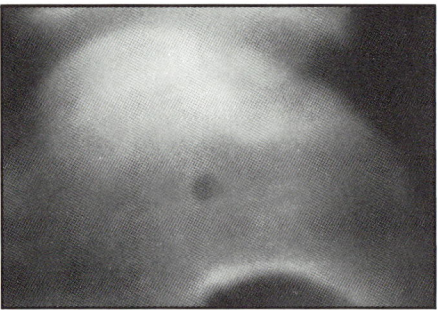

Figure 10-5. R.M. This lateral x-ray shows a lesion of osteochondritis dissecans, as seen in the midportion of the talar dome. It was inaccessible for arthroscopic drilling from the usual portals. This was the first case of transmalleolar drilling, and was done prior to use of the distraction method.

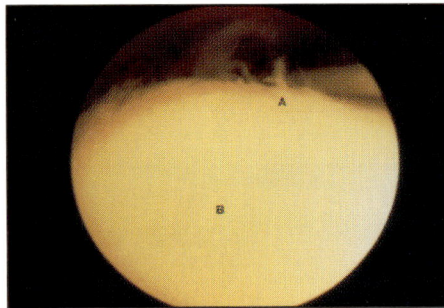

Figure 10-6. R.M. This is an arthroscopic view, with the ankle in extreme plantar flexion, showing that this intact lesion has difficult accessibility for drilling from routine portals. A, margin of osteochondritis lesion; B, dome of talus.

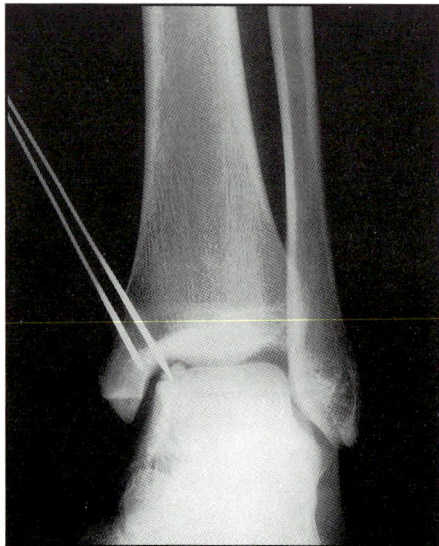

Figure 10-7. R.M. This is an AP x-ray view showing two .062 Kirschner wires drilling the lesion via the transmalleolar approach.

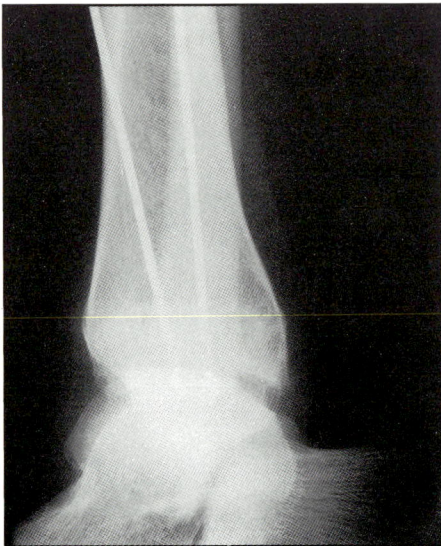

Figure 10-8. R.M. This lateral x-ray view shows the wire placement for transmalleolar drilling.

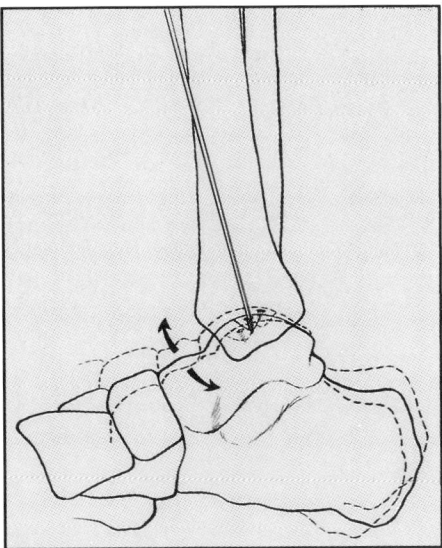

Figure 10-9. R.M. This diagram shows that two parallel wires are used for drilling. The ankle is flexed and extended. Several drill holes can be made (up to eight in number). In this case, there were six.

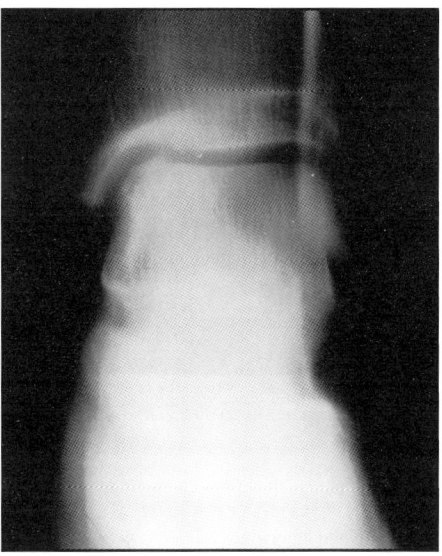

Figure 10-10. R.M. An AP x-ray view after two months. Healing is seen.

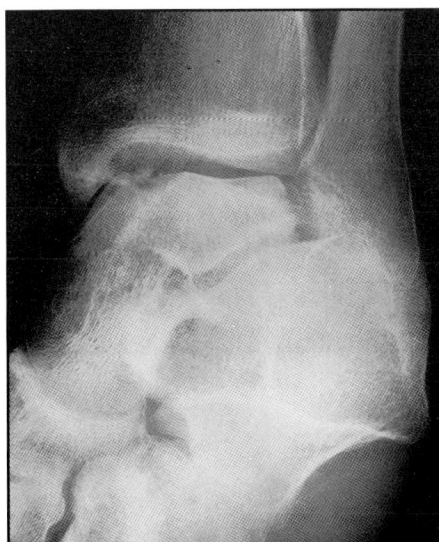

Figure 10-11. M.K. This AP x-ray shows a lesion that appears to be separated. At arthroscopy the lesion was intact, and only normal articular cartilage was seen in that area.

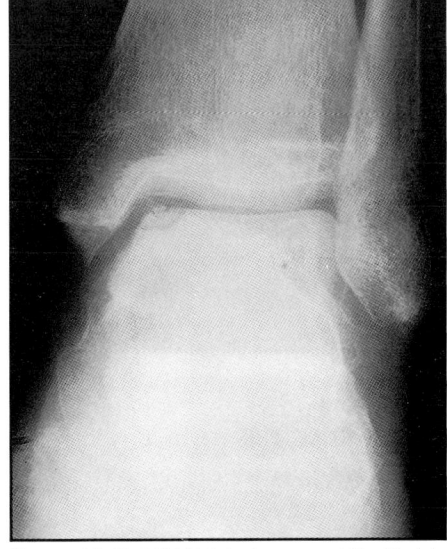

Figure 10-12. M.K. This lesion was drilled inside with the use of an arthroscopic anterior cruciate ligament guide. Healing occurred ten weeks later, according to clinical judgement, and remained healed one year later. The x-ray did not show complete evidence of healing. This is typical of about 50% to 60% of such cases. The x-ray picture will probably persist indefinitely, despite clinical healing.

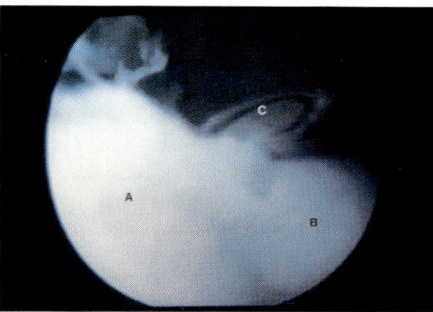

Figure 10-13. J.P. This is a video arthroscopic view. The above lesion appeared intact at x-ray but was not intact at arthroscopy, since the articular cartilage over the lesion was different in texture and color. This was easily lifted with a needle. A, separated osteochondritis lesion; B, dome of talus; C, tip of hypodermic needle.

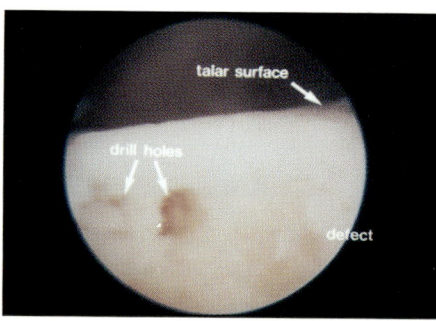

Figure 10-14. J.P. This postoperative 35mm arthroscopic view shows the lesion after reconstruction and drilling in the right ankle.

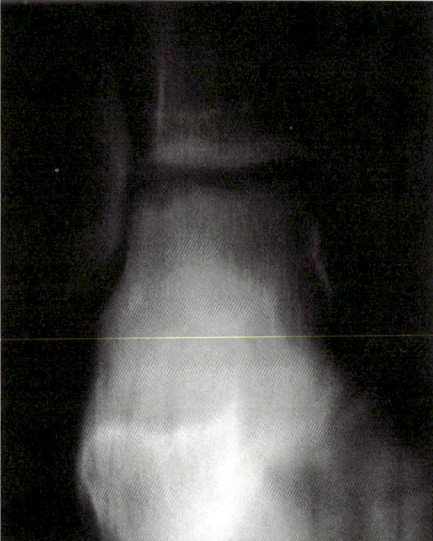

Figure 10-15. J.G. This is an AP x-ray view of an "intact lesion" of the medial talus.

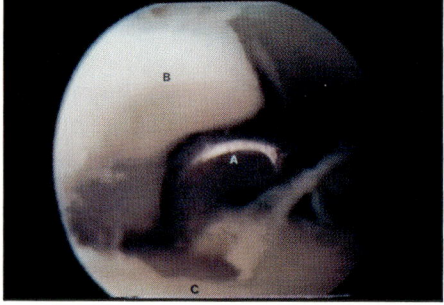

Figure 10-16. J.G. This video arthroscopic view shows the probe lifting off the diseased articular cartilage at the site of the lesion. A, probe; B, flap of cartilage; C, base of lesion.

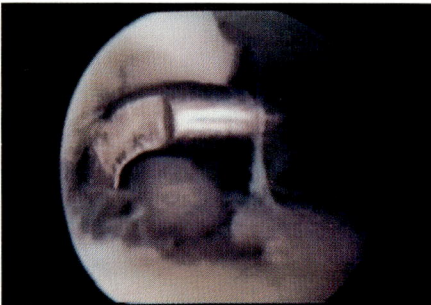

Figure 10-17. This is another arthroscopic video view showing the bed of the lesion.

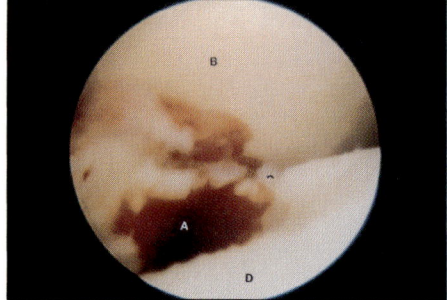

Figure 10-18. J.G. This 35mm arthroscopic view, after reconstruction, shows bleeding following release of the tourniquet. This is important, as it confirms that there was sufficient abrasion and drilling. A, fresh bleeding; B, plafond; C, reconstructed crater; D, dome of talus.

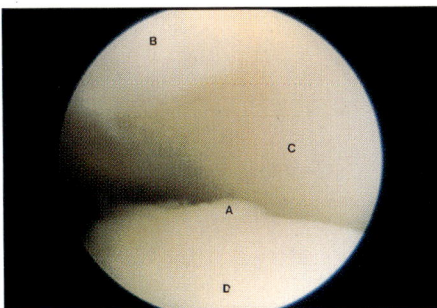

Figure 10-19. R.R. This is a 35mm arthroscopic preoperative view of osteochondritis dissecans with a separated lesion. Note the small fragment that can barely be seen at this point with distraction. A, separated osteochondritis lesion; B, plafond; C, medial malleolus; D, dome of talus.

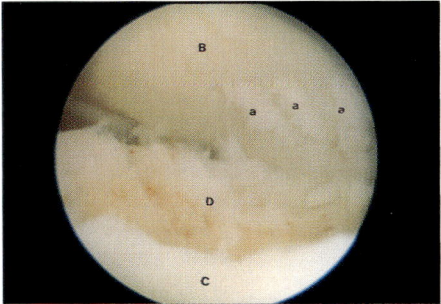

Figure 10-20. R.R. This is a 35mm arthroscopic view after reconstruction and drilling. Note the three transmalleolar drill holes (A). B, plafond; C, dome of talus; D, reconstructed defect.

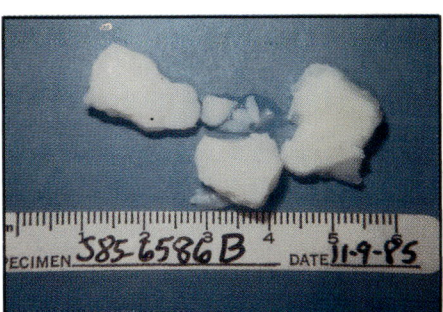

Figure 10-21. R.R. The specimen that was removed.

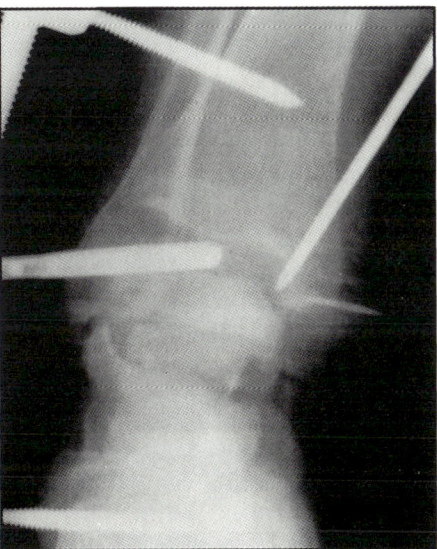

Figure 10-22. R.R. An AP x-ray view showing placement of wires for drilling.

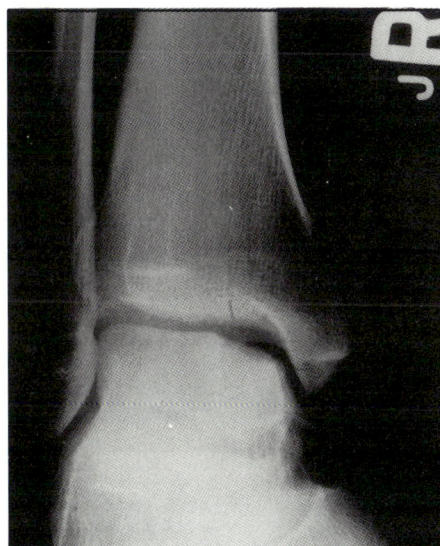

Figure 10-23. E.E. An AP x-ray with a large lesion of the right ankle. This 34-year-old man had osteochondritis dissecans treated by an arthrotomy and curettage three years before being seen by the author. A large loose body was removed at the time. According to the operative report, drilling was not done. The patient continued to have symptoms.

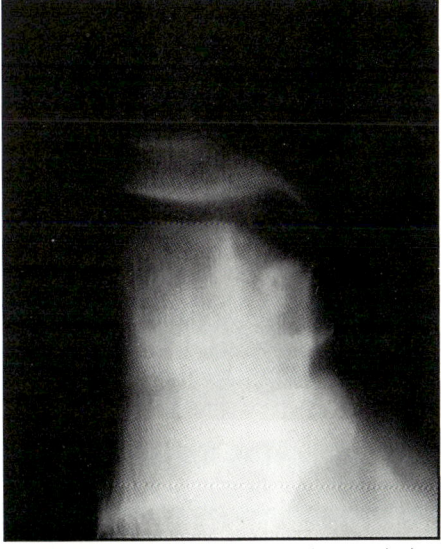

Figure 10-24. E.E. A tomogram shows a lesion much larger and more extensive than the routine x-ray.

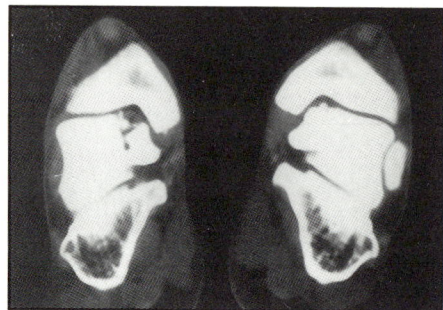

Figure 10-25. E.E. The same lesion demonstrated by a CT scan. This technique is reported to be superior to the tomogram, as far as showing the location and extent of the lesion for preoperative planning.

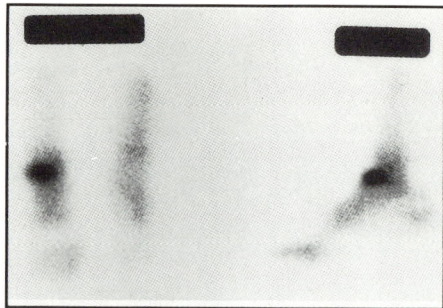

Figure 10-26. E.E. A bone scan of the same case shows a moderate uptake of the right ankle, as well as a weak uptake of the left talus. Multiple x-ray views of the left ankle showed a very small osteochondritis lesion.

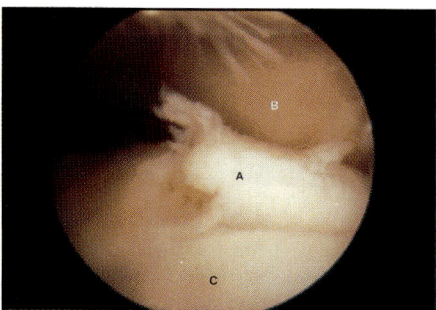

Figure 10-27. E.E. This video arthroscopic view shows the poor quality of fibrocartilage that filled in the defect. A flap of tissue (A) was easily lifted from this lesion with a probe; B, medial malleolus; C, dome of talus.

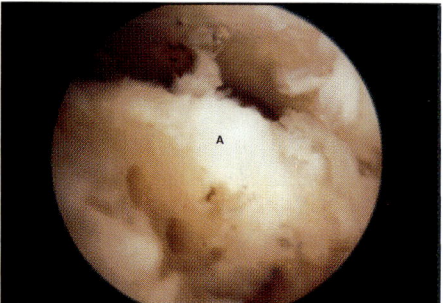

Figure 10-28. E.E. A video arthroscopic view after reconstruction. Note the drilling was also done in the posterior direction to get at that portion of the lesion (A) underlying good bone and articular cartilage.

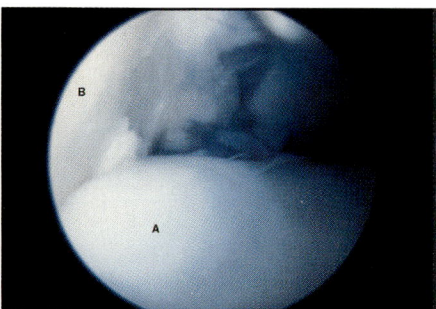

Figure 10-29. W.R. This 35mm arthroscopic view shows another lesion of the medial talar dome that "appears intact." The diseased articular cartilage is outlined and is white in appearance after the injection of the methylene blue dye. A, Osteochondritis lesion; B, medial malleolus.

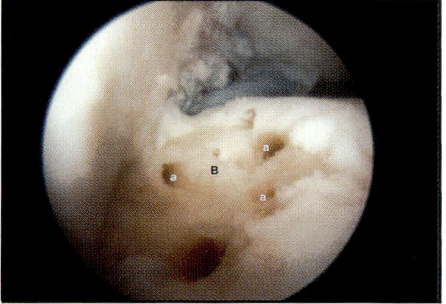

Figure 10-30. W.R. A 35mm arthroscopic view of the same lesion above after reconstruction. A, drill holes; B, lesion.

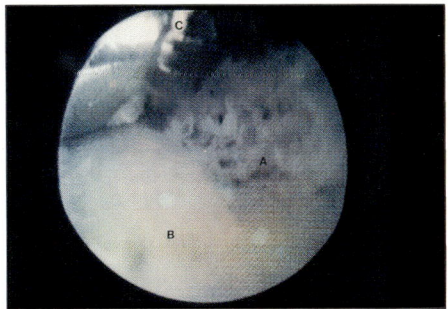

Figure 10-31. B.W. This is a video arthroscopic view of a reconstructed crater (A) (osteochondritis dissecans) in the medial dome of the talus (B). Note the arthroscopic abrader (C) in the upper left corner.

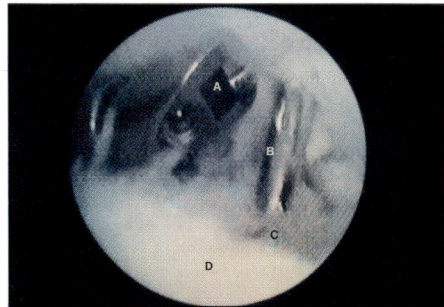

Figure 10-32. B.W. The same view as above, showing the 70 degree oblique arthroscope (A) (posterolateral portal) in the upper left corner and an .062 Kirschner wire (B) through the medial malleolus and into the crater (C) for drilling the base. D, dome of talus.

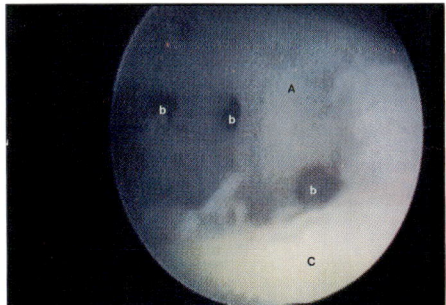

Figure 10-33. B.W. This is another video arthroscopic view of the same crater (A) through the 70 degree oblique arthroscope inserted through the posterolateral portal. B, drill holes; C, dome of talus.

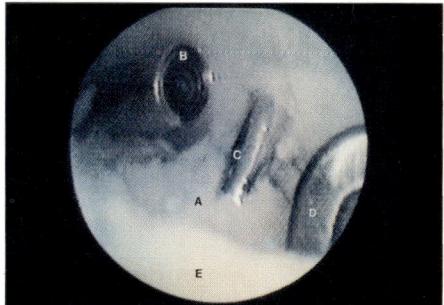

Figure 10-34. B.W. A video arthroscopic view of the same crater as above. (A), the medium sized (2.5mm) arthroscope (B) in the upper left corner (posterolateral portal). The Kirschner wire (C) in the middle and the probe (D) in the lower right corner are shown. E, dome of talus.

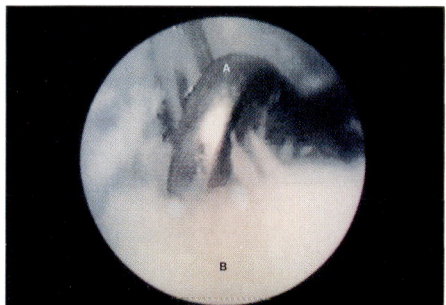

Figure 10-35. B.W. A video arthroscopic view through the midsized arthroscope (2.5mm) from the posterolateral approach. The probe (A) is shown lifting the posterior surface of the crater and demonstrating an additional significant amount of loose diseased cartilage (B) that was not appreciated from the anterolateral approach.

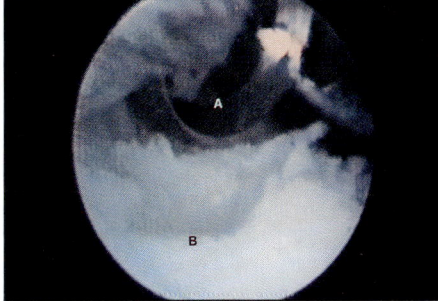

Figure 10-36. B.W. A view through the 2.5mm arthroscope (posterolateral probe), showing a curette (A) removing the remaining loose cartilage. B, margin of deficit.

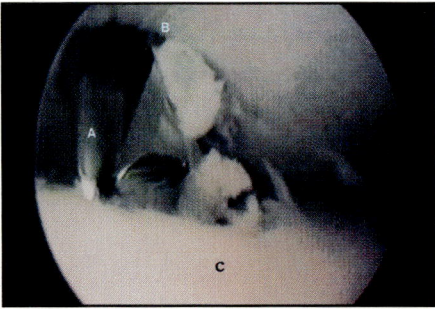

Figure 10-37. C.S. This arthroscopic video view shows the drill tip creating an adequate channel for instrumentation in a lesion located far posterior. Several graduated drill sizes can be used (or a cannulated reamer as an alternate method). A, drill; B, defect; C, dome of talus.

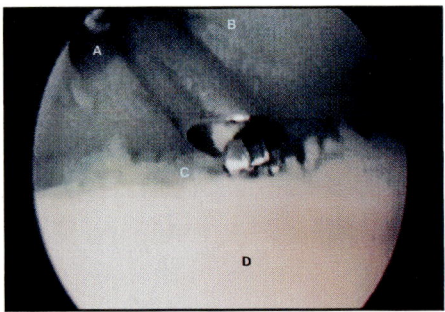

Figure 10-38. C.S. This arthroscopic video view shows the abrader for preparing the base and trimming the margin of the lesion. A, channel through medial malleolus; B, abrader; C, defect; D, dome of talus.

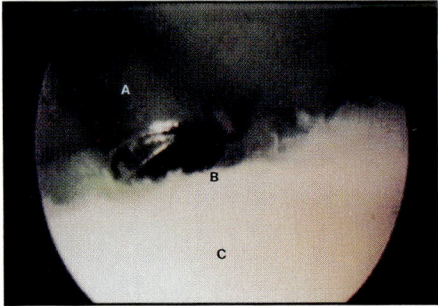

Figure 10-39. C.S. Same arthroscopic video view as above. Note: A, 2.5mm intermediate arthroscope protruding through the defect. B, margin of defect. C, dome of talus.

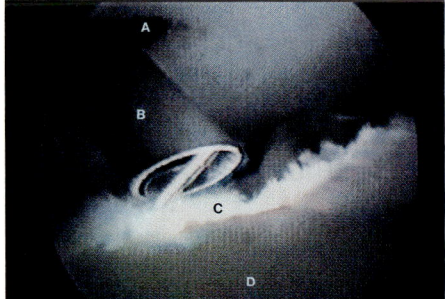

Figure 10-40. C.S. Same arthroscopic video view as above. The light cable is now changed to the small arthroscope.

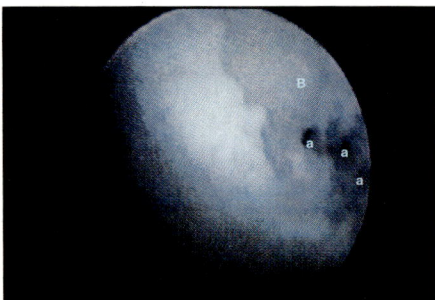

Figure 10-41. C.S. View of above lesion through 2.5 arthroscope via transmalleolar channel.

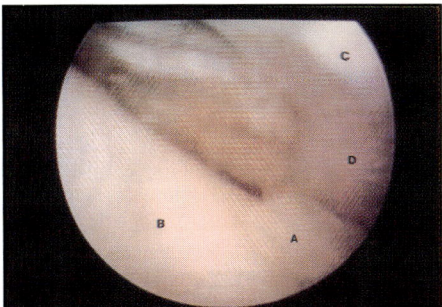

Figure 11-1. J.K. This is a video arthroscopic view of a partially separated chondral lesion (A) of the medial talar dome (B) in the right ankle. C, plafond; D, medial malleolus.

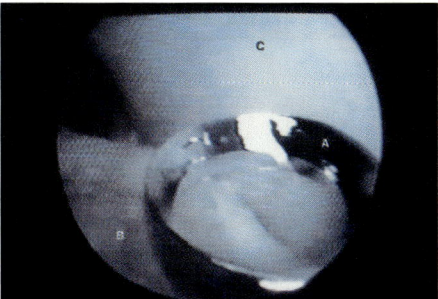

Figure 11-2. J.K. A video arthroscopic view of the above lesion after debridement. A curette (A) is shown removing the fibrous tissue from the base. B, lesion; C, medial malleolus.

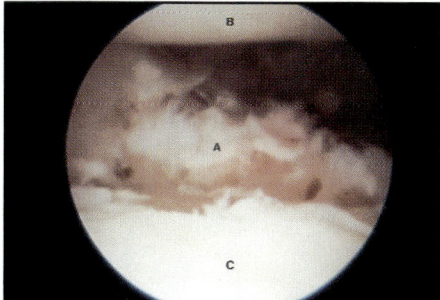

Figure 11-3. C.D. A 35mm arthroscopic view shows another case of a chondral lesion of the talar dome after debridement. A, debrided lesion; B, plafond; C, dome of talus.

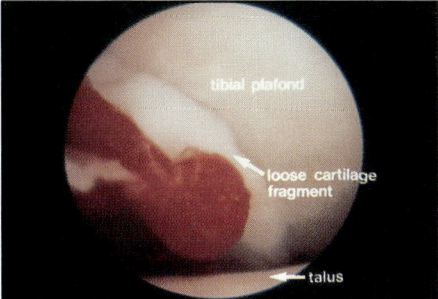

Figure 11-4. L.P. This is a 35mm arthroscopic view of a lesion of the lateral tibial plafond with a loose body in place in the right ankle.

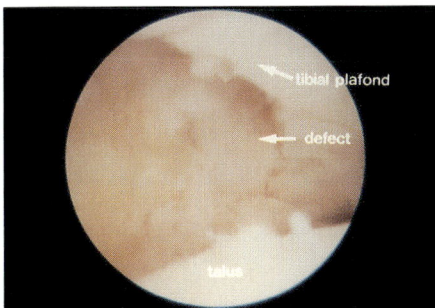

Figure 11-5. L.P. A 35mm arthroscopic view of the above lesion after the loose fragment was removed and the crater was debrided, abraded, and drilled.

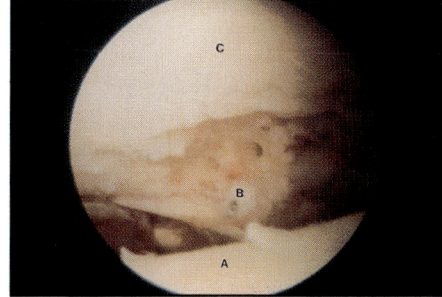

Figure 11-6. A.B. A 35mm arthroscopic view of another chondral lesion of the lateral tibial plafond after reconstruction (A) talus (B) lesion (C) platond.

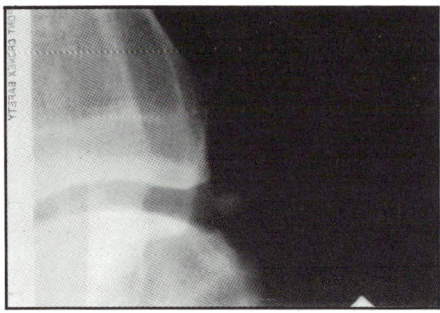

Figure 11-7. F.R. This lateral x-ray shows a single osteochondral loose body in the posterior compartment of the ankle joint in the left ankle.

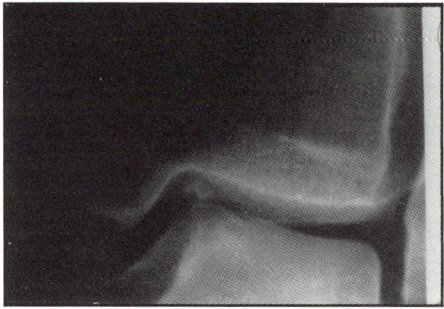

Figure 11-8. F.R. This AP x-ray shows the loose body in the posterior portion of the medial talomalleolar joint.

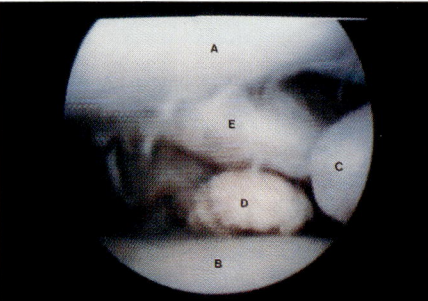

Figure 11-9. F.R. A video arthroscopic view, with the plafond (A) shown above and the dome (B) below. The osteochondral loose body (C) is at the right. Another small chondral loose body (D) is at center. The transverse tibiofibular ligament (E) can be seen in the posterior compartment.

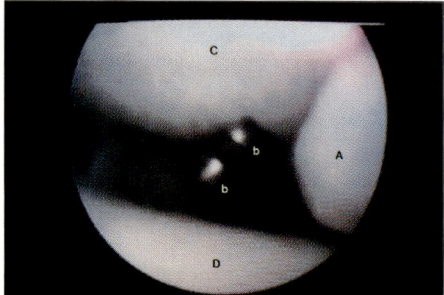

Figure 11-10. F.R. A video arthroscopic view of same case. The loose body (A) has moved to the medial side of the ankle joint proper. The grasping forceps (B) is shown about to remove the fragment. C, plafond; D, dome of talus.

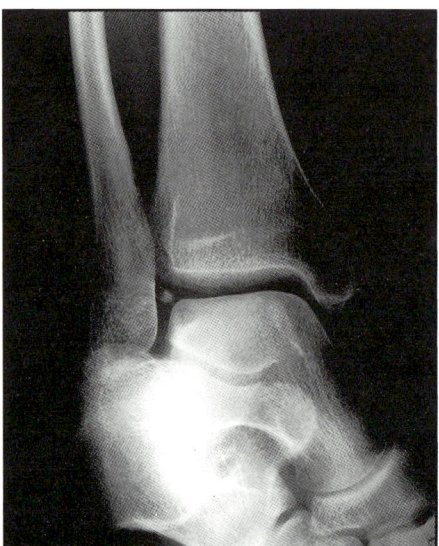

Figure 11-11. T.T. An AP x-ray shows an osteo-cartilagenous loose body in the posterior portion of the lateral talomalleolar joint in the right ankle. This fragment did not move on cineradiographic examination.

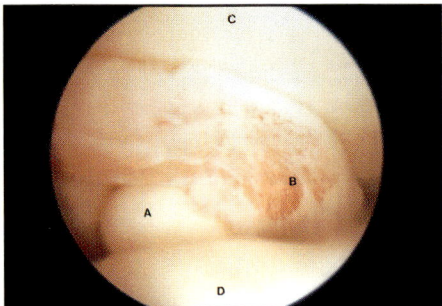

Figure 11-12. T.T. A 35mm arthroscopic view of the same patient. This shows a loose body (A) in the center of the picture held by a "sling" of synovial impingement tissue (B). The loose body was easily dislodged with a probe and removed with a grasping forceps. C, plafond; D, dome of talus.

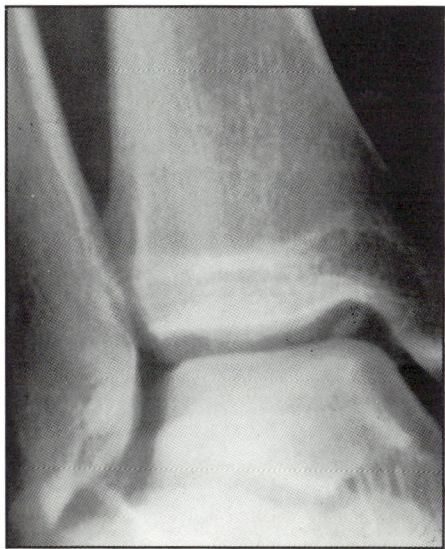

Figure 11-13. M.N. An AP x-ray. This view (only) showed a symptomatic loose body in the posteromedial corner of the right ankle joint. It was fixed or not movable on video record motion studies.

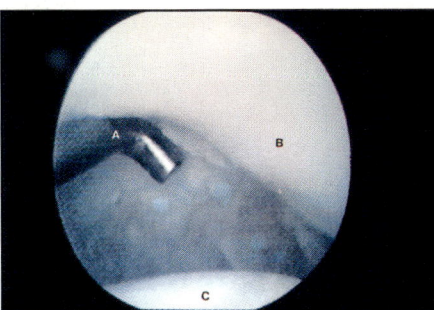

Figure 11-14. M.N. A video arthroscopic view of complete exploration with a probe (A) from combined anterior approaches and with the ankle distracted. The exploration failed to locate the lesion. B, medial malleolus; C, dome of talus.

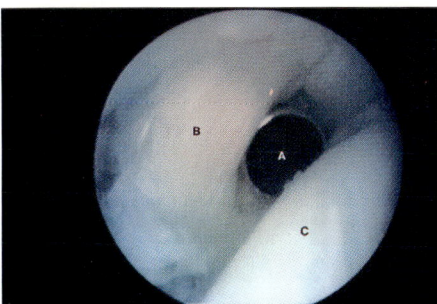

Figure 11-15. M.N. This video arthroscopic view shows the cannula (A) of the intermediate or 2.5mm arthroscope inserted from the posterolateral portal. Note the transverse tibiofibular ligament (B) above and the talus (C) below.

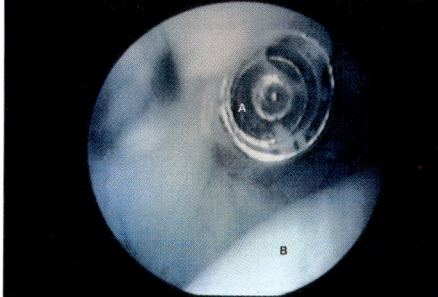

Figure 11-16. M.N. A video arthroscopic view. The same as above with the lens system in the cannula. A, lens of arthroscope; B, dome of talus.

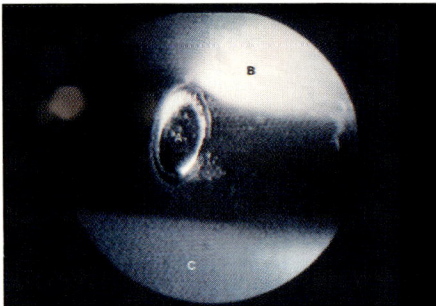

Figure 11-17. M.N. A video arthroscopic view of the same case as above. The light cable has been switched from the large arthroscope in the anterolateral portal to the 2.5mm arthroscope in the posterolateral portal. A, lens of arthroscope; B, plafond; C, dome of talus.

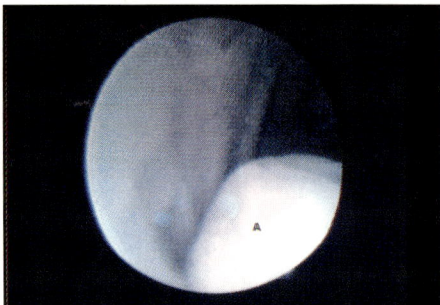

Figure 11-18. M.N. A video arthroscopic view of the same case. This view is through the smaller arthroscope in the posterolateral corner of the talus. (Larger 5mm arthroscopes can be inserted from this approach just as well in most cases.) A, posteromedial dome of talus.

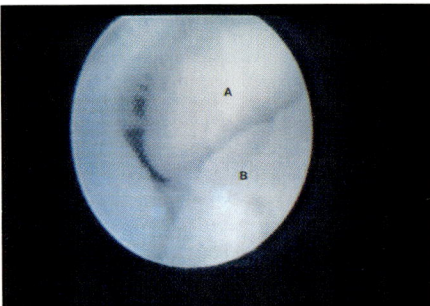

Figure 11-19. M.N. Another video arthroscopic view of the same case. The loose body (A) is located as the tip of the 2.5mm arthroscope which is manipulated about the posteromedial corner of the ankle joint. B, posteromedial dome of talus.

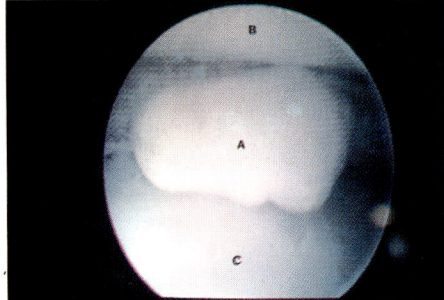

Figure 11-20. M.N. This is a 5mm video arthroscopic view from the anterolateral portal. The loose body (A) was manipulated from the position shown in Figure 11-19 to the mid talocrural joint. It was then easily removed by triangulation from the anterior approaches. B, plafond; C, dome of talus.

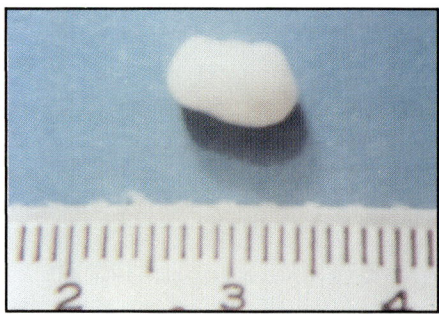

Figure 11-21. M.N. The specimen is shown in relation to the scale to be 3mm x 4mm x 8mm.

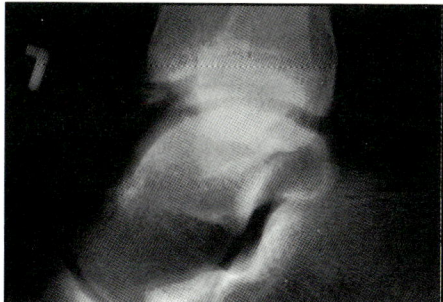

Figure 11-22. N.L. This lateral x-ray of the left ankle shows an anterior impingement lesion (osteophyte) in a professional football kicker.

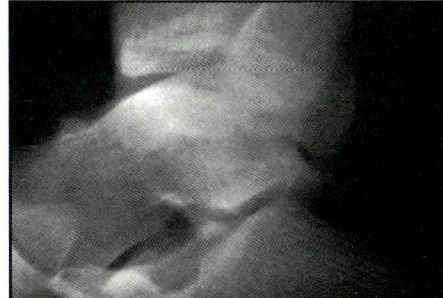

Figure 11-23. N.L. The same view after a successful arthroscopic excision.

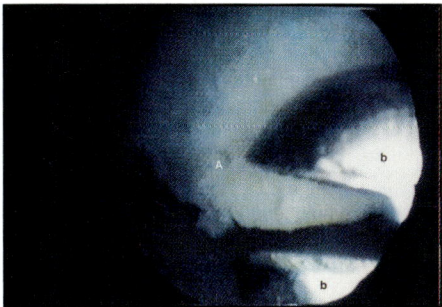

Figure 11-24. N.L. This video arthroscopic view shows the osteophyte (A) being removed with a downbiting pituitary rongeur (B).

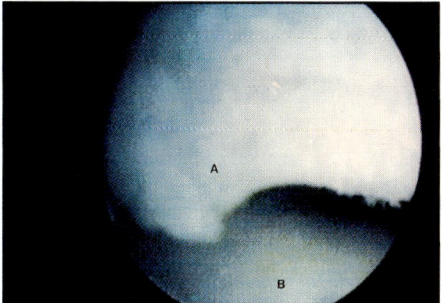

Figure 11-25. N.L. This is a video arthroscopic view of the same case after a portion of the lesion has been removed. A, osteophyte; B, dome of talus.

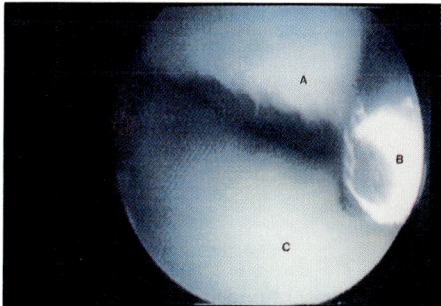

Figure 11-26. N.L. Another video arthroscopic view in the same case shows the remainder of the osteophyte (A) excised with a small osteotome (B). C, dome of talus.

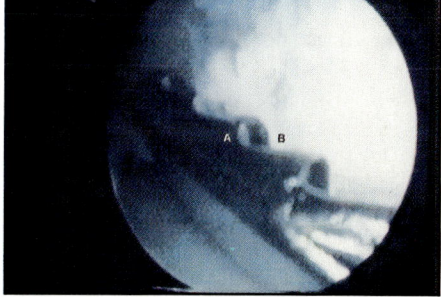

Figure 11-27. N.L. A final TV arthroscopic view. The rasp (A) is used to smooth the remaining margin of the anterior tibia. B, osteophyte.

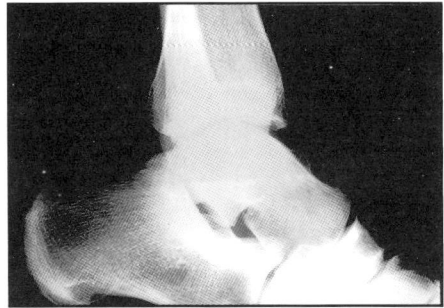

Figure 11-28. R.B. This lateral x-ray shows a similar anterior impingement lesion.

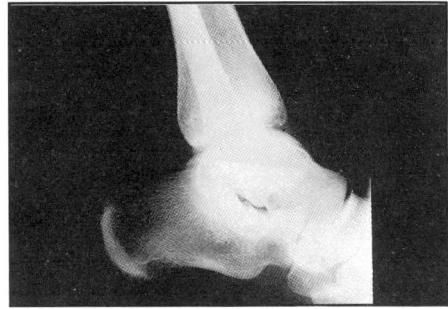

Figure 11-29. R.B. The same view after successful arthroscopic excision.

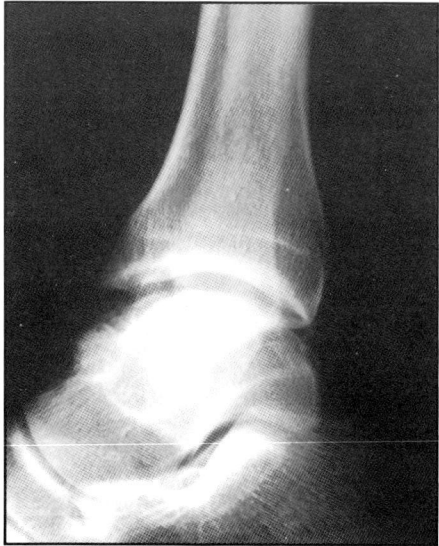

Figure 11-30. J.W. A patient with symptomatic anterior impingement lesion on lateral x-ray in the left ankle.

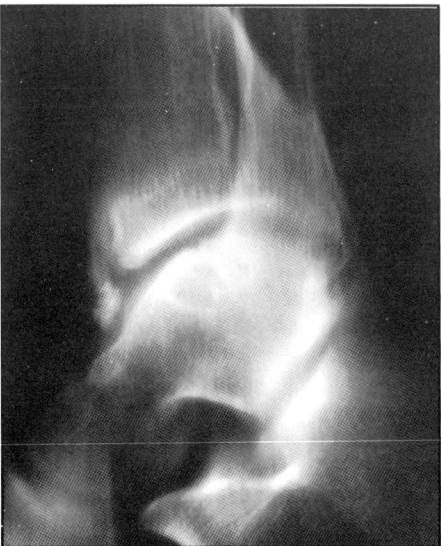

Figure 11-31. J.W. These lateral tomograms showed the lesion to be a loose body adherent to the synovium and a defect of the tibial plafond. Two loose bodies were removed at arthroscopy, and the defect was reconstructed.

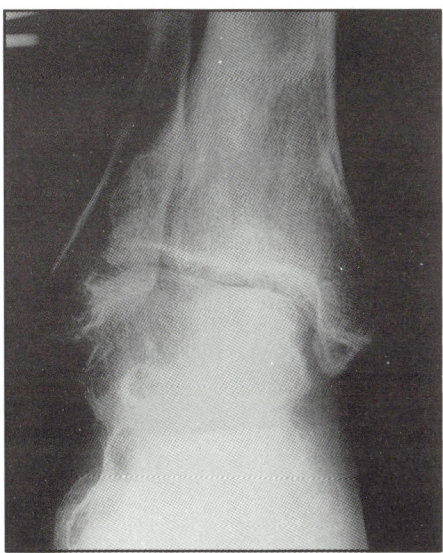

Figure 11-32. P.P. An AP x-ray of a "painful, stiff" right ankle with early degenerative changes.

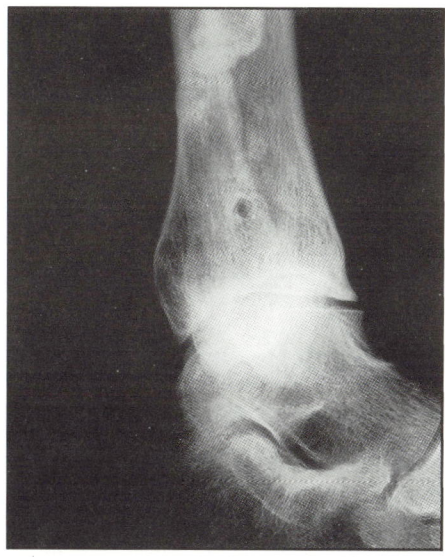

Figure 11-33. P.P. This lateral x-ray of the same case shows early narrowing of the joint line with a large osteophyte of the anterior tibial ridge and the neck of the talus.

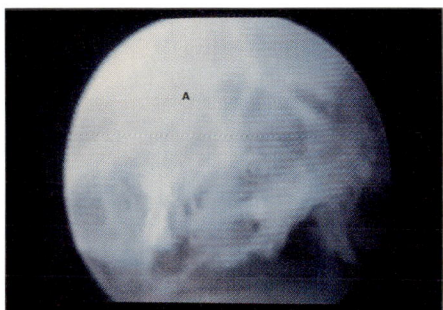

Figure 11-34. P.P. A TV arthroscopic view of chondromalacia of the plafond (A).

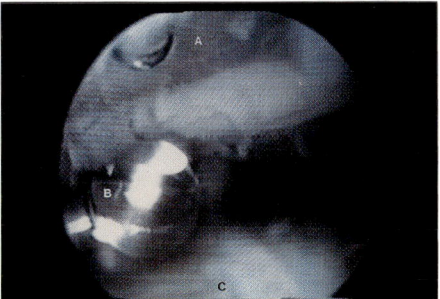

Figure 11-35. P.P. A TV arthroscopic view after the chondromalacia was probed and debrided. A chondral defect (A) was then apparent. The abrader (B) is shown. C, dome of talus.

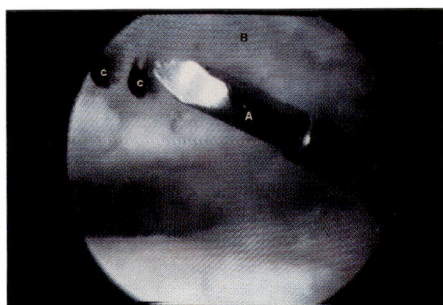

Figure 11-36. P.P. A TV arthroscopic view showing the defect being drilled with an .062 Kirschner wire (A) through a small cannula. B, crater; C, drill holes.

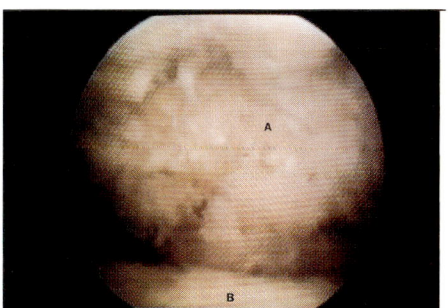

Figure 11-37. P.P. A TV arthroscopic "second look" was done. Fibrocartilage of fair quality (A) was found. B, dome of talus.

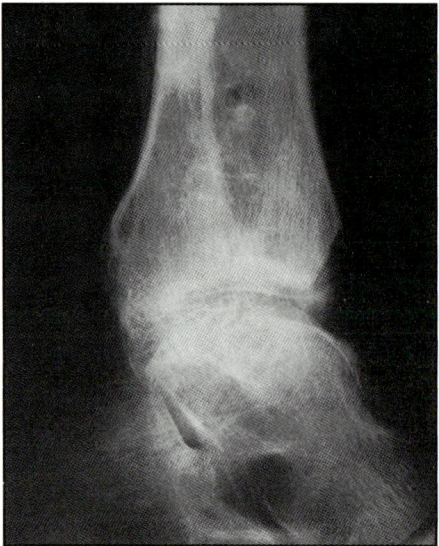

Figure 11-38. P.P. This lateral x-ray shows the same case five months later. An arthrotomy was done, utilizing a medial and lateral approach to excise the symptomatic osteophyte.

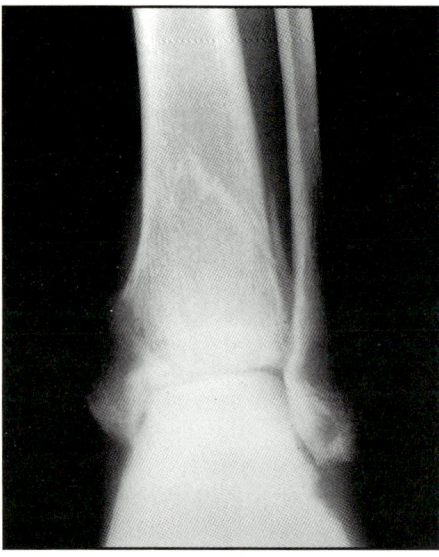

Figure 11-39. M.R. This is an AP x-ray of a displaced trimalleolar fracture of the left ankle (Ferkel).

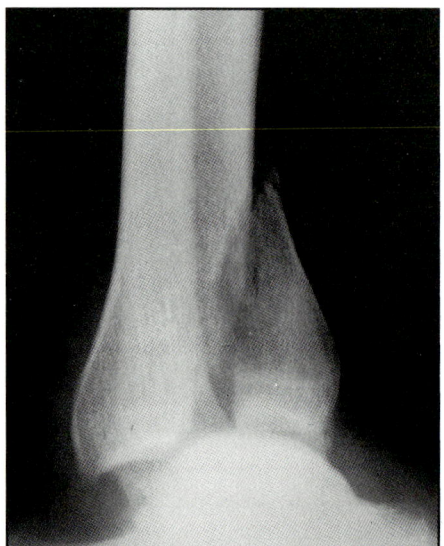

Figure 11-40. M.R. This is a lateral x-ray of the same ankle fracture (Ferkel).

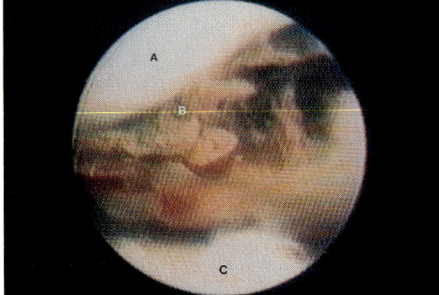

Figure 11-41. M.R. A video arthroscopic view of the plafond (A) portion of the fracture before reduction. The early callous (B) was excised with a curette. C, dome of talus. (Ferkel).

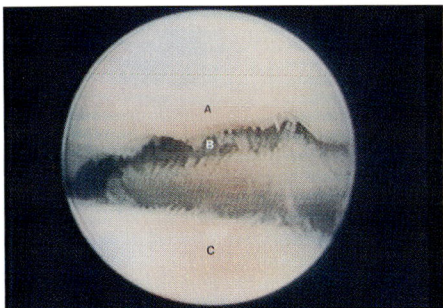

Figure 11-42. M.R. A video view of the same case after the callous was excised. A, plafond; B, fracture; C, dome of talus. (Ferkel).

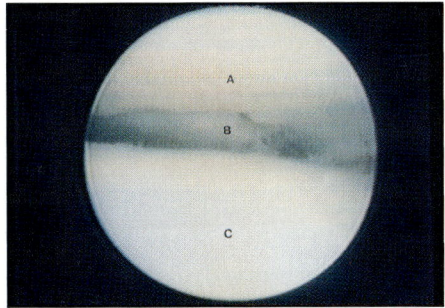

Figure 11-43. M.R. The same view after a perfect hairline reduction under arthroscopic control. A, plafond; B, fracture; C, dome of talus. (Ferkel).

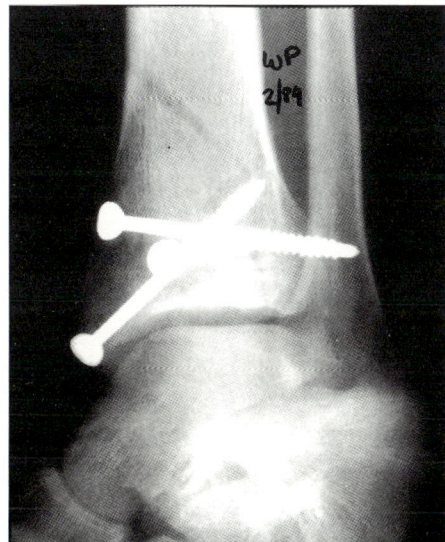

Figure 11-44. M.R. An AP x-ray of the above case after reduction and fixation (Ferkel).

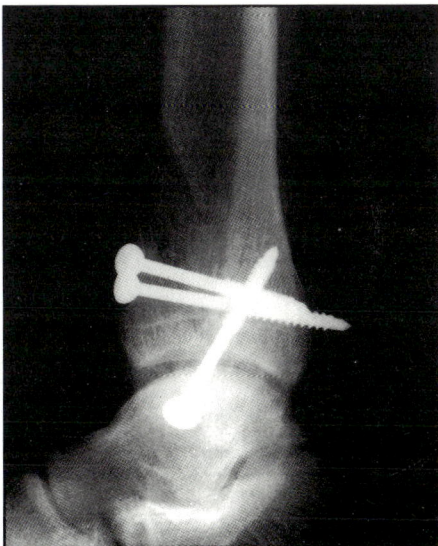

Figure 11-45. M.R. A lateral x-ray after reduction and fixation (Ferkel).

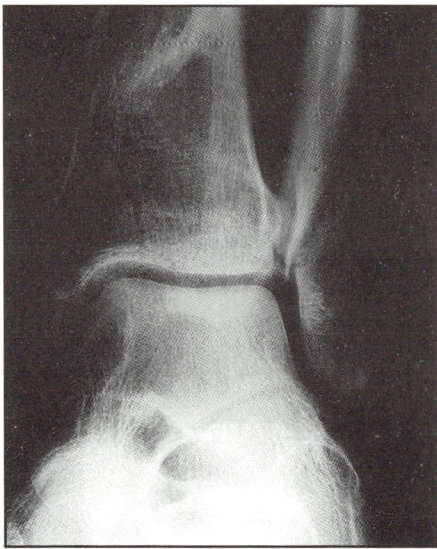

Figure 11-46. T.F. An AP x-ray of an oblique fracture of the fibula extending into the lateral talomalleolar joint.

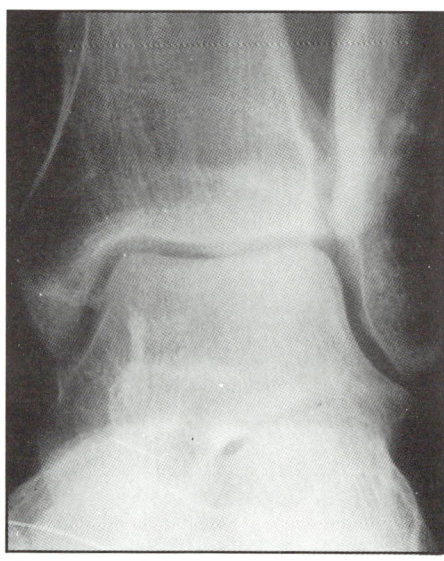

Figure 11-47. T.F. The same case with the fracture healed. Pain and tenderness persisted on the lateral side of the ankle joint.

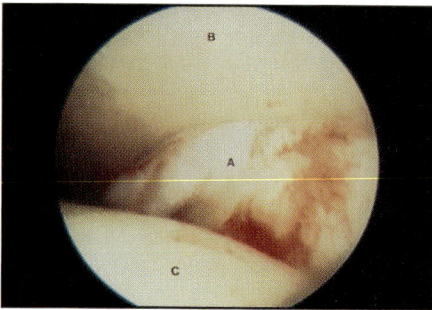

Figure 11-48. T.F. This 35mm arthroscopic view shows a lateral impingement lesion (A) with some osteocartilagenous tissue at the interarticular site of the fracture. B, plafond; C, dome of talus.

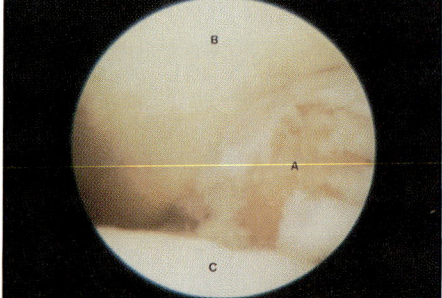

Figure 11-49. T.F. This is a postoperative 35mm arthroscopic view. A, excised lesion; B, plafond; C, dome of talus.

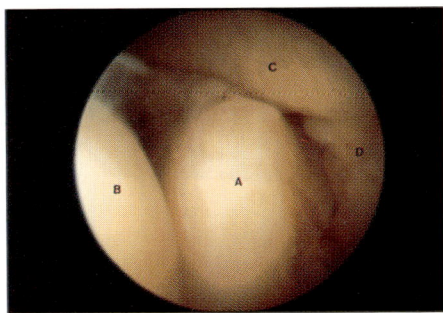

Figure 11-50. P.L. A 35mm arthroscopic view of a symptomatic posttraumatic osteocartilagenous lesion (A) in the lateral talomalleolar joint. Excision arthroscopically afforded some relief. B, talus; C, plafond; D, fibula.

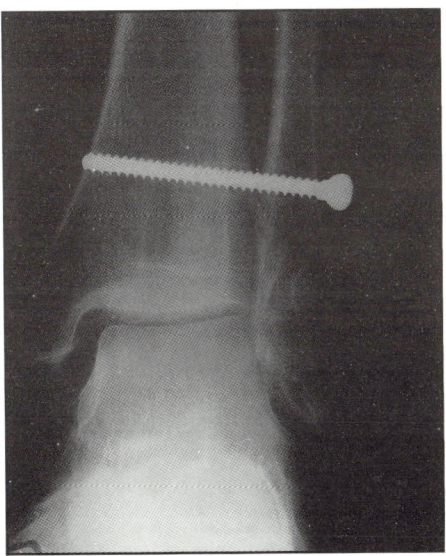

Figure 11-51. R.W. An AP x-ray after an open reduction of a fracture of the distal fibula, which was then fixed to the tibia with an OA screw. Symptoms persisted months after healing. This view shows the residual dyastasis of the medial talomalleolar joint. Symptoms were relieved with arthroscopic excision of the synovial, capsular, and ligamentous tissues.

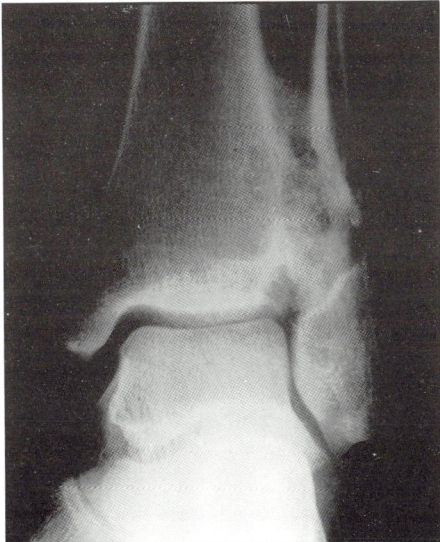

Figure 11-52. J.B. This 17-year-old girl had a synostosis of the tibiofibular joint after multiple open surgical procedures. Pain persisted in the lateral talomalleolar part of the ankle. At arthroscopy a large amount of organized fibrocartilagenous tissue was removed from the superior portion of the lateral talomalleolar joint, resulting in symptomatic relief.

CHAPTER 12

ARTHROSCOPIC TIBIOTALAR ARTHRODESIS

Craig D. Morgan, M.D.

In general, the arthroscopic technique to be described recreates a previously reported open method of tibiotalar arthrodesis.[1] Equipment necessary to perform this procedure includes: an image intensifier and radiolucent operating table, a 30 degree 4mm arthroscope with camera and TV/video equipment, a highspeed motorized suction abrader and shaver, and an external fixation apparatus with distraction capability.

Operative Technique

The patient is positioned supine and generally anesthetized on a standard operating table with a radiolucent foot and ankle extension. A sandbag is placed under the buttock of the operative limb to avoid external rotation of the leg during the procedure. After routine prep and drape from the proximal tibia to the toes, a proximal thigh tourniquet is inflated, following Esmarch exsanguination.

The ankle and foot are suspended on a large cloth bump placed behind the posterior aspect of the midcalf, which allows access to the posterolateral aspect of the ankle. Following this, an external fixation halfframe with distraction capability is applied medially that is used to distract the tibiotalar articulation, allowing for adequate arthroscopic visualization. Mechanical distraction of the tibiotalar joint is an absolute necessity; without this step, there is insufficient space to allow for adequate visualization, as well as placement of operating instruments. Distraction is applied, using a standard Acufex distractor device attached to two three-sixteenth inch diameter Schanz halfpins placed under image intensification through small 3mm stab wounds.

The proximal pin is placed in the medial "bare" area of the tibia, approximately one and one-half inches above the ankle joint and is driven through both tibial cortices such that the pin is placed parallel to the tibiotalar articulation. In a similar fashion, the distal pin is driven from medial to lateral into the body of the talus, beginning from a skin puncture placed just inferior and slightly anterior to the tip of the palpable medial malleolus. This medial entry point for the distal pin will place the pin near the center of the dorsiflexion-plantar flexion rotation axis of the talar dome and will allow the surgeon to plantar flex and dorsiflex the talus during the procedure, despite significant distraction of the joint. Care should be taken to avoid placing the distal pin behind the medial malleolus for fear of injury to the posterior tibial tendon or the neurovascular structures (Figures 12-1 and 12-2). Once proper pin placement is achieved, approximately one-quarter inch of distraction is applied using the Synthes turnbuckle distraction attachment. Distraction is maintained throughout the procedure.

Three standard arthroscopic portals are used: the anterolateral, anteromedial, and posterolateral. With the arthroscope placed from a standard anterolateral portal, the amount of necessary distraction is assessed. Once good visualization is achieved, a large-bore cannula for fluid inflow is introduced through a posterolateral portal under direct arthroscopic visualization from in front. Following this, a standard diagnostic arthroscopy is then performed. Next, using a motorized arthroscopic abrader in a systematic fashion, taking care to maintain the normal bony contour of the talar dome and tibial plafond (i.e., talar convexity and tibial concavity), the articular surfaces of the tibial plafond, talar dome, and medial and lateral talar-malleolar surfaces are debrided of all remaining hyaline cartilage and subchondral bone, thus exposing viable cancellous bone (Figure 12-3). Care should be taken not to "square off" the surfaces.

Debridement of the most posterior aspect of the talus and posterior malleolus is accomplished by maximally plantar flexing the foot. Occasionally, use of a ringed curette with a 15 degree bend 1.5cm from the working end allows debridement of the hyaline cartilage in this region where the

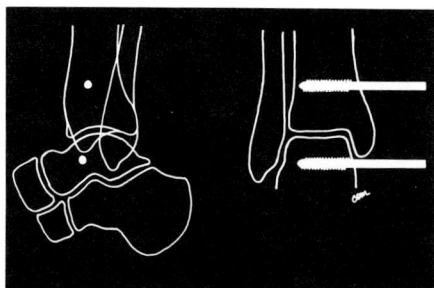

Figure 12-1. A schematic illustration of tibial and talar external fixation pin placement.

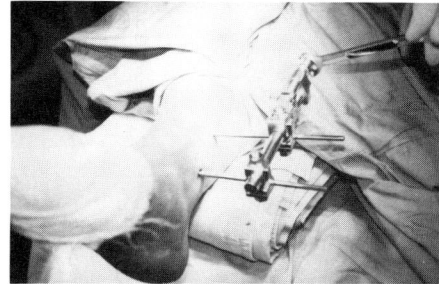

Figure 12-2. A medial halfframe applied to a right ankle. Note the turnbuckle distraction device at the superior aspect of the frame.

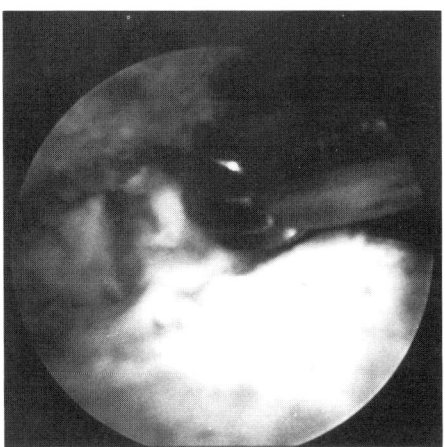

Figure 12-3. An intraarticular picture of exposed cancellous bone created by motorized abrader, with the tibial plafond above and the talus below.

motorized abrader sometimes will not reach. In general, the medial half of the debridement process is done with the arthroscope placed anterolaterally and the abrader placed anteromedially. Conversely, the lateral half of the debridement process is done with the arthroscope placed anteromedially and the abrader anterolaterally. The final step in the debridement process includes placing the arthroscope posterolaterally to visualize the usual large anterior tibial "lip osteophyte". This must be removed or it will block adequate reduction of the talar dome convexity into the concavity of the tibial plafond. This osteophyte is removed using the motorized abrader from in front, while visualizing from behind.

Once viable cancellous bone is visualized surrounding the fusion area, the distraction device is released and the fusion surfaces are reduced under image intensification by upward displacement of the hindfoot and dorsiflexion of the forefoot to a neutral position. With the talus held in this position, internal fixation is obtained with two screws placed percutaneously, one from the medial distal tibial metaphysis and one from the distal fibula metaphysis into the body of the talus.[1] These screws angle anteriorly, approximately 40 degrees, to gain maximum purchase into the talus without entering the subtalar joint (Figures 12-4 and 12-5). Confirmation of the fusion reduction and screw placement is then done using the image intensifier or permanent x-rays.

All portals are then closed with a single #4-0 Nylon stitch and the Schanz external fixation pins are removed. Next, the ankle is immobilized in a well padded short-leg cast. The patient is kept nonweight bearing for six weeks postoperatively, followed by an additional six weeks in a short-leg walking cast.

Indications

An arthroscopic approach to ankle fusion versus open surgery is felt to be advantageous in patients with systemic problems leading to an increased risk of poor wound healing—such as hemophilia, rheumatoid arthritis, diabetes

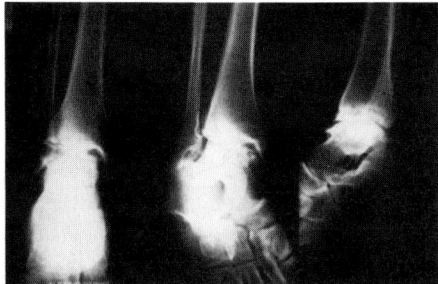

Figure 12-4. Preoperative radiographs of a right ankle with severe Factor VIII deficient hemophiliac arthropathy.

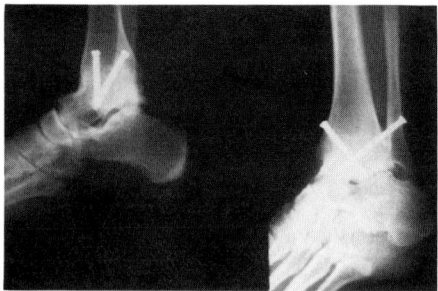

Figure 12-5. Two-year postfusion radiographs of the same ankle.

mellitus, peripheral vascular occlusive disease, or longterm corticosteroid use.

Contraindications

This arthroscopic approach is felt to be contraindicated in patients with severe varus or valgus deformity of the tibiotalar articulation (greater than 15 to 20 degrees). In these patients only an open approach offers adequate and accurate bone removal to allow for correction of severe deformity.

This procedure is quite tedious and requires great attention to details. With this in mind, the surgeon should be well versed in all arthroscopic techniques, and, in particular, should have substantial experience in small joint (nonknee joint) arthroscopy prior to attempting the procedure.

Clinical Experience

I have successfully fused three ankles with this technique (two hemophiliacs and one posttraumatic arthritic) without complications. In one additional case, I was unable to reduce the fusion after the debridement step and completed the fusion with an arthrotomy. In this case, dense scarring in the medial and lateral talomalleolar spaces was blocking the reduction. In retrospect, this scarring probably could have been "cleaned out" arthroscopically.

At the time of this writing, I am aware of six additional successful fusions, using similar arthroscopic techniques.[2,3] In this group, one complication of a pseudoaneurysm of the dorsalis pedis artery occurred, secondary to use of an anterocentral portal.[2] For this reason, use of an anterocentral approach is not recommended.

References

1. Morgan CD, et al.: Long Term Results of Tibiotalar Arthrodesis. J Bone & Joint Surg 67(A):546-50, 1985.
2. Glick J: Personal Communication, 1986.
3. Patel D: Personal Communication, 1986.

CHAPTER 13

STAPLING REPAIR FOR CHRONIC LATERAL ANKLE INSTABILITY

Richard B. Hawkins, M.D.

With the advent of better technique and equipment for ankle arthroscopy, new options have become available for treating common orthopedic problems. Such an example is the use of arthroscopic staples to reattach a chronically elongated lateral capsule and the anterior talofibular ligament to the abraded surface of the lateral talus.

Since 1982, we have offered this procedure to patients with a history of chronic lateral ankle instability brought on by repeated inversion sprain injuries that are usually sports related. Most patients prefer an outpatient arthroscopic procedure to traditional procedures involving incisions, such as the Watson-Jones or similar lateral ankle reconstructions.

The purpose of this chapter is to present the elements of the technique as it has been developed to date. Longterm followup studies of large numbers of patients are not yet available so we emphasize to patients that arthroscopic ankle stapling is an alternative whose ultimate place in the orthopedic armamentarium is not yet known.

The Clinical Problem

Lateral ankle sprains are among the most common of all athletic injuries. Most sprains heal uneventfully with traditional conservative treatment. Some patients, however, develop chronic instability symptoms, usually after suffering several moderate to severe lateral ankle sprains. The patient with clinically significant lateral ankle instability will describe a progression of events over months or even years, indicating increasing laxity of the ankle.

Minor provocations, such as stepping off a curb or down a stair, can lead to a significant inversion injury to the ankle.

Frequently, it is possible to detect a positive anterior drawer test caused by rupture or laxity of the anterior talofibular ligament. The examiner's hand, grasping the heel, can slide the entire foot forward at the tibiotalar joint, using the opposite hand to anchor the leg. Many of these patients will show an increased amount of "talar tilt" on radiographs. When inversion stress is applied, the talus appears to tilt out or invert from the lateral aspect of the tibia. Usually the results of this test are quite subtle, unless the calcaneofibular ligament and anterior talofibular ligaments are both torn.

Arthroscopic reconstructive surgery has advanced significantly in the past few years with the introduction of the Instrument Makar Ligamentous and Capsular Repair System. This system, consisting of small 5.5mm or 6.7mm staples, an inserter-extractor and placement cannula, has allowed the successful repair of torn anterior cruciate ligaments in the knee and reattachment of glenohumeral ligaments in the shoulder for treatment of chronic instability.

For more than four years we have performed lateral ankle stabilizations under arthroscopic control, using the arthroscopic stapling system. In these cases, the anterior talofibular ligament and contiguous capsule are plicated into an abraded area on the adjacent medial surface of the talus with the small 5.5mm staple under arthroscopic visualization.

Biomechanics

The ankle, because of its geometry and ligamentous support, is a supple and strong joint for locomotion. Nevertheless, it is prone to injury from a variety of mechanisms, most commonly from an excessive plantar flexion and inversion stress. In this position, the anterior talofibular ligament is aligned nearly parallel to the long axis of the tibia.[10,17] In plantar flexion and inversion, the anterior talofibular ligament is loaded by inversion and internal rotary movements.[3,7] A number of biomechanical studies of the ankle have measured increased ankle motion after sectioning of the various ligaments.[1,2,11,12,16] The results showed that injury to the anterior talofibular ligament allows anterior and medial displacement of the talus. Inversion of the talus was also observed with the foot in excessive plantar flexion.

Other studies using radiographic techniques have shown that the anterior talofibular ligament does not contribute very much to the varus tilt of the talus,[4,17] unless injury has also occurred to the canlcaneofibular ligament.[8,18] Still another experimental study of the ankle under loaded conditions showed significant increases in rotation without simultaneous increase in varus angulation after dividing the anterior talofibular ligament.[14] Another important biomechanical study[11] found the anterior talofibular ligament to be a primary stabilizer of the ankle, indicating that it provides significant resistance to varus tilt of the talus in all positions of flexion. The authors noted that because the increased motions of the talus are relatively small after sectioning only the anterior talofibular ligament, many ankles that are chronically symptomatic following ankle injury may have increased talar instability secondary to insufficiency of the anterior talofibular ligament, which is essentially undetectable by clinical or radiographic evaluation.

Many open surgical procedures have been utilized for reconstructing the lateral ligament in cases of chronic instability of the ankle. Elmslie,[5] Evans,[6] Good, et al.,[9] Seftom, et al.,[19] Ottosson,[15] Storen,[20] and Watson-Jones,[21] have all described techniques that often involve using the peroneus brevis for a lateral reefing. Levy[13] has added a synthetic reinforcement band. The arthroscopic stapling procedure is an alternative method with the same goal of lateral reefing or stabilization.

Arthroscopic Technique

All of our arthroscopic ankle procedures are done as outpatient surgeries under general anesthesia, using a thigh tourniquet, as in all extremity surgery, and a legholding device applied to the midcalf. It is important to avoid undue pressure over the proximal calf near the fibular neck, which could lead to peroneal palsy. For ankle ligament reconstruction we have found portal placement to be exceedingly important. An 18-gauge needle is used to establish an anteromedial portal just anterior to the saphenous vein and medial to the anterior tibial tendon. As saline is instilled through a 30cc syringe, the ankle dorsiflexes. Another 18-gauge needle localizes an anterolateral portal through which the Storz 2.7mm arthroscope is introduced.

Although a lateral 4mm arthroscope can be used to visualize the ankle joint, we have found it technically difficult to gain exposure in the lateral gutter near the tip of the fibula. A 3mm water inflow cannula is then inserted in the anteromedial portal already established by the first 18-gauge needle. The saline bag is suspended at least one meter above the ankle, providing a sufficient head of pressure for distention of the joint for the surgical procedure. If viewing appears compromised by inadequate distention, the saline bag can be inserted into the Zimmer Aries pressure device. The foot pedal attached to the device can then be used to increase the pressure in the saline bag until viewing on the monitor is improved, taking care not to exceed about 100mm on the associated pressure gauge.

The diagnostic part of the procedure then commences. Patients with chronic lateral instability of the ankle will often show a relative laxity or "ballooning" of the entire lateral capsule and anterior talofibular ligament when viewed from an anterolateral portal. Cadaver dissection is an important prerequisite to performing this procedure and will reveal that the lateral capsule and anterior talofibular ligament are contiguous structures that are in reality quite thin in comparison to the thick deltoid ligament medially. An increased synovitis is often present in patients with chronic lateral instability. Loose bodies are not uncommon. Frequently, articular cartilage defects are seen at the medial corner of the joint where the corner of the talus has struck the tibia at the medial aspect of the plafond during a subluxation or inversion stress. Articular cartilage loose bodies may be aspirated through the arthroscope in these cases or retrieved with grasping forceps.

Arthroscopic stapling repair for chronic lateral instability is simply a shortening or tightening of the lateral capsule and anterior talofibular ligament (Figure 13-1). A 6mm or 8mm diameter area on the vertical surface of the talus is abraded about 1cm anterior to the tip of the lateral malleolus. An accessory portal is established with an 18-gauge needle about 1cm distal to the anterolateral portal used for the arthroscope. The powered instruments can then be introduced at about a 45 degree angle to the area on the vertical surface of the talus that is to be abraded. The abrasion is done with the Dyonics Small Joint System. A 2.8mm abrader tip is used to denude articular cartilage down to bleeding bone (Figure 13-2). The 2.8mm synovial resector is then used to remove soft tissue and debris so that a smoothly tapered surface is created slightly larger than the staple. Finally, a small sized arthroscopic staple from the Instrument Makar Ligament and Capsular Repair System is inserted from a fourth portal chosen so that the staple will enter the talus at a right angle. The two tines of the staple surround and gather capsule and ligament tissue and are lined up with the prepared bed on the talus.

The foot is brought to the neutral position to allow sufficient tightening of the lateral structures (Figure 13-3). After insertion of the staple with a mallet, the inserter-extractor device is unscrewed (Figure 13-4). Since the space at the site of the staple insertion is virtually obliterated, viewing on the monitor at this point becomes impossible. Therefore, as a final step, the arthroscope can be withdrawn and then reinserted in the fourth portal to allow direct visualization of the staple itself with secured ligament tissue within the staple neck. As a final check, an anteroposterior and lateral radiograph can be obtained to verify the correct position of the staple.

No sutures are used. All portals are left to close secondarily for minimal scarring, after infiltrating them with 0.25 percent bupivacaine and epinephrine solution to minimize postoperative bleeding and discomfort. Typical postoperative radiographs are shown in Figure 13-5. A bulky dressing is applied, followed by a posterior plaster splint and an elastic bandage. Five

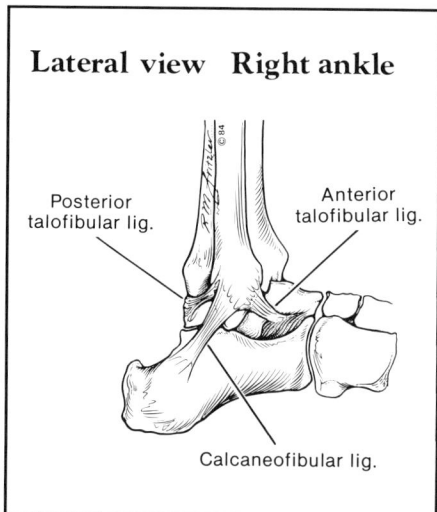

Figure 13-1. A lateral view of the right ankle, demonstrating ligamentous structures.

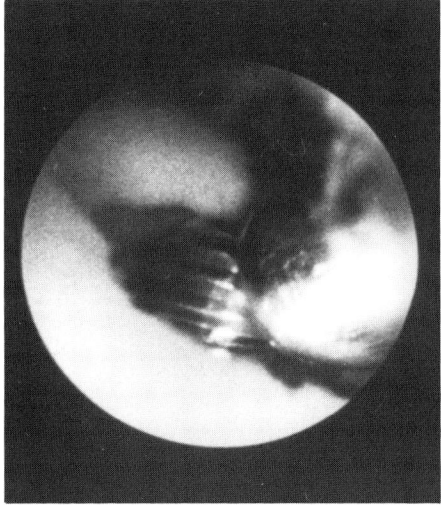

Figure 13-2. An abrader preparing the talus for stapling. (Courtesy of Dr. R. Lundeen.)

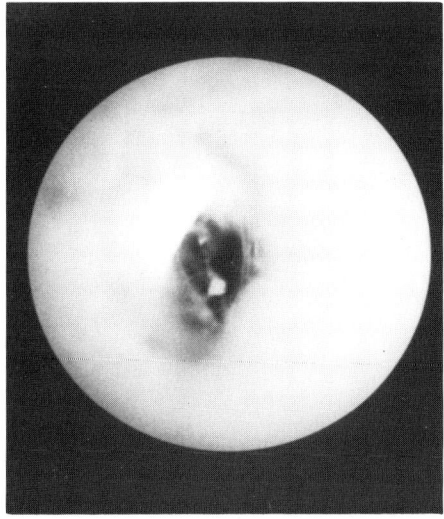
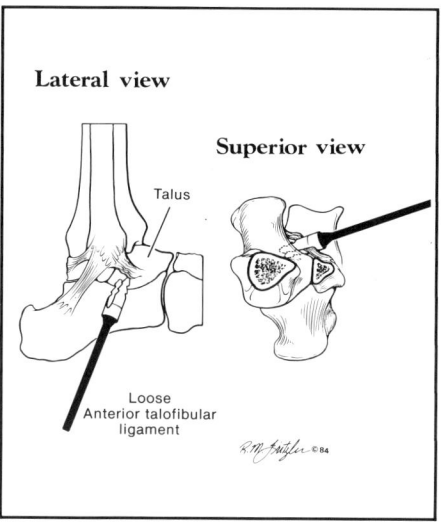

Figure 13-3. A staple securing the lateral ligamentous structure to the talus. (Courtesy of Dr. R. Lundeen.)

Figure 13-4. The lateral view (left) and the superior view (right) of staple insertion.

days later the initial dressings are removed in the the outpatient department and a fiberglass walking cast is applied. The patient is encouraged to discard crutches when comfortable, usually at about ten days. After six weeks the cast is removed and range of motion and strengthening exercises are begun. An elastic pull-on support or aircast is recommended for sports during the first few months.

Initially, we carried out "second look" arthroscopies at three months and removed the staple. We found that an intense fibrous tissue reaction had occurred, correcting the lateral ankle instability quite adequately. In fact, viewing into the lateral gutter was difficult. Extraction of the staple requires a cutdown incision over the staple head. The staple can be so imbedded in bone, ligament, and scar that it is difficult to find and remove. In cases done over the past three years, the staples have been left in place, to be removed only if they should cause symptoms.

Results

Followup evaluations in more than two dozen patients have been quite gratifying, showing greatly improved stability and allowing patients to return to normal activities and functional levels, including sports. No patient has yet wished to have traditional surgery for lateral reconstruction. Longest followups are now more than four years. Inversion stress radiographs have shown marked improvement, although not to the level of the normal side. For example, one patient had a preoperative stress radiograph showing 18 degrees of talar tilt, compared to five degrees on the normal ankle. Three months postoperative he was asymptomatic and the inversion stress radiograph on the operated ankle showed nine degrees of talar tilt.

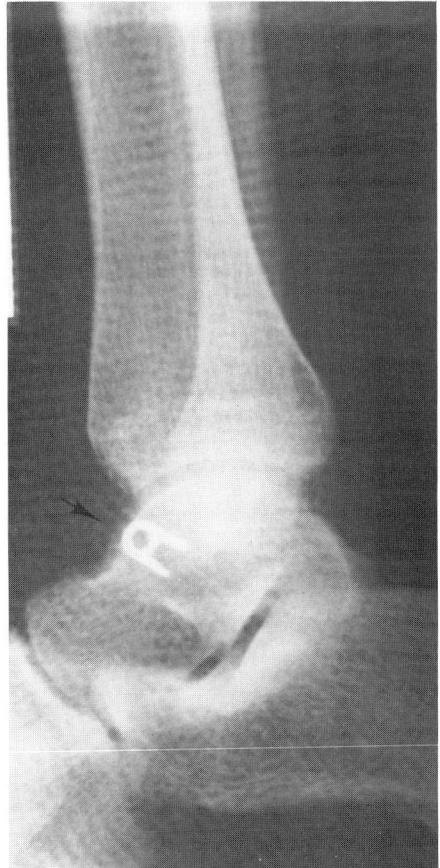 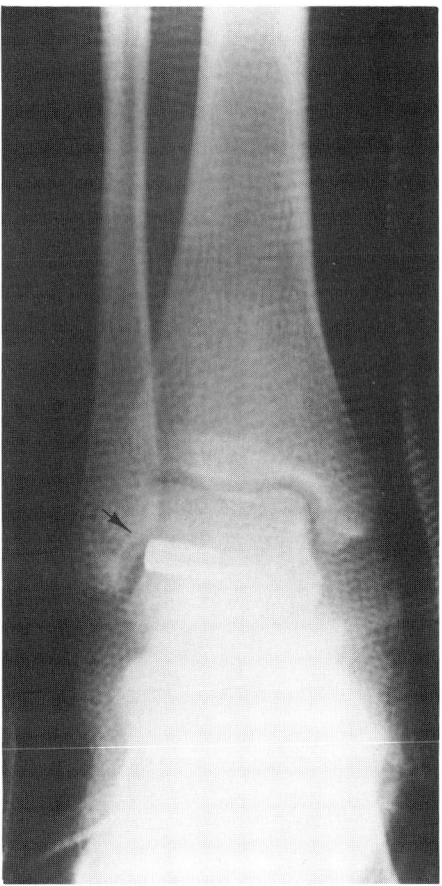

Figure 13-5A. Postoperative lateral radiograph showing position of the staple.

Figure 13-5B. Postoperative anterior/posterior radiograph showing position of the staple.

Complications

As clinical experience grows with any surgical experience, there inevitably arises the occasional complication. Most complications can be avoided by careful and meticulous technique. In one patient, the staple was inadvertently placed at an angle so that the tines entered the subtalar joint. This was recognized in subsequent films. The staple was removed after three months, at which point healing had occurred. No further symptoms have developed.

In another patient, just the opposite problem occurred; the radiographs suggested the staple tines were close to protruding into the tibiotalar joint. Again, the staple was removed electively. The "second look" arthroscopy did not reveal any injury to articular cartilage of the talus.

One patient in this series underwent a second procedure due to recurrent instability. Nine months after a successful stapling for chronic instability brought on by repeated softball injuries, he was again injured while playing softball. Because of the recurrent symptoms, a "second look" arthroscopy was carried out. The staple was firmly in position in the side of the talus, but all the soft tissues were avulsed from around it. The staple was removed, a wider abrasion was performed, and a new staple inserted. He has now been free of complaints for two more years, and continues to play softball with an ankle support.

Another complication reported to us by a colleague involved a patient who developed inability to extend his little toe after the stapling repair. This complication was treated by staple removal and apparently was related to fixation of a portion of the extensor mechanism in the repair.

Case Report

D.A., a 28-year-old self-employed building contractor, presented with a complaint of chronic "giving out" of the left ankle. The first injury had occurred during high school with an inversion stress during running. Marked swelling of the lateral ankle had lasted nearly a week. Over ten years he had had innumerable episodes of ankle sprain, associated with transient disability, but his major complaint was a feeling of instability of the ankle. His work as a contractor involved walking on uneven terrain, so he had learned to avoid perching on roofs for fear his ankle would give out. Clinical evaluation confirmed a 3+ anterior drawer test and varus instability. Stress radiographs showed a talar tilt of 16 degrees, compared to four degrees in his normal ankle (Figure 13-6).

At the time of outpatient arthroscopy of the ankle, loose cartilage debris was aspirated from the joint and a surface defect was seen at the medial plafond on the tibial surface. A stapling reconstruction was carried out. Eighteen months later he was clinically asymptomatic. In fact, he has

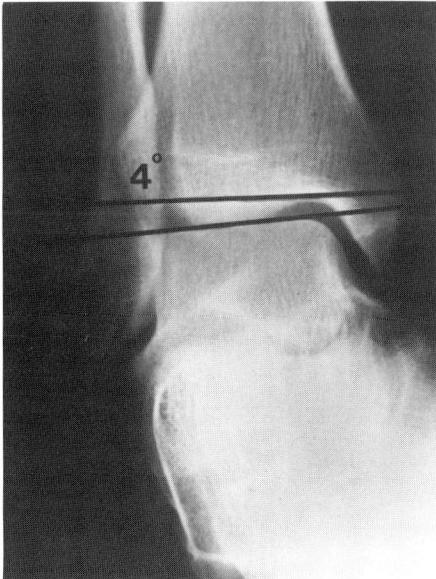

Figure 13-6A. Stress radiograph showing the four degree talar tilt of the normal right ankle.

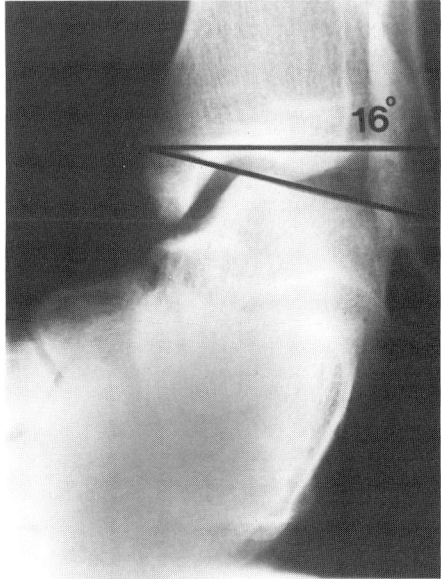

Figure 13-6B. Stress radiograph showing the 16 degree tilt of the unstable left ankle.

resumed climbing on roofs and playing softball, using a soft elastic brace for support. His followup stress radiograph showed improvement, despite persistence of varus instability of 11 degrees, indicating probable damage to the calcaneofibular ligament.

Summary

We have presented a preliminary report on a limited number of patients with chronic lateral instability of the ankle treated with arthroscopic stapling reconstruction. As stated, the longest followups are four years, so the results over the longterm are not yet known. Early results have been quite encouraging, however, with improved functional stability of the ankle. Only one patient in more than two dozen has had recurrent instability that required more surgery. He returned with a history of additional sports trauma.

The principle of secure fixation of ligaments to exposed bone surfaces with staples is a well accepted and effective technique familiar to orthopedists for many years. What is changing is that microsurgical techniques can now be adapted to common orthopedic problems. As in most outpatient arthroscopic procedures, there is a high degree of patient acceptance of the procedure. Discomfort is minimal and some patients have not even filled their prescriptions for analgesic medication. The period of disability is relatively short and rehabilitation rapid. As in most arthroscopic surgical procedures, instruments of the correct size are most important, as is precise surgical technique. The key to success is careful forethought, planning, and teamwork.

References

1. Anderson, KJ, LeCocq JD: Operative Treatment of Injury to the Fibular Collateral Ligament of the Ankle. Am J Bone & Joint Surg 36:825-832, 1954.
2. Anderson, KJ, LeCocq JD, LeCocq EA: Recurrent Anterior Subluxation of the Ankle Joint. Am J Bone & Joint Surg 34:853-860, 1952.
3. Brostrom L: Sprained Ankles I: Anatomic Lesions in Recent Sprains. Acta Chir Scand 128:483-495, 1964.
4. Chrisman OD, Snook GA: Reconstruction of Lateral Ligament Tears of the Ankle: An Experimental Study and Clinical Evaluation of Seven Patients Treated by a New Modification of the Elmslie Procedure. Am J Bone & Joint Surg 51:904-912, 1969.
5. Elmslie RC: Recurrent Subluxation of the Ankle Joint. Am Surg 100:364-367, 1934.
6. Evans DL: Recurrent Instability of the Ankle: A Method of Surgical Treatment. Proc R Soc Med 46:343-344, 1953.
7. Freeman MAR: Instability of the Foot After Injuries to the Lateral Ligament of the Ankle. Br J Bone & Joint Surg 47:669-677, 1965.
8. Glasgow M, Jackson A, Jamieson AM: Instability of the Ankle After Injury to the Lateral Ligament. Br J Bone & Joint Surg 62:196-200, 1980.

9. Good JC, Jones MA, Livingstone BN: Reconstruction of the Lateral Ligament of the Ankle. Injury 7:63-65, 1975.
10. Inman VT: The Joint of the Ankle. Baltimore, Williams & Wilkins, 1976, pp. 3-10.
11. Johnson EE, Markolf KL: The Contribution of the Anterior Talofibular Ligament to Ankle Laxity. Am J Bone & Joint Surg 65:81-88, 1983.
12. Leonard MH: Injuries of the Lateral Ligament of the Ankle: A Clinical and Experimental Study. Am J Bone & Joint Surg 31:373-377, 1949.
13. Levy M: Newly Modified Evans Operation Enables Immediate Mobilization. Orth Rev 15:73-77, 1986.
14. McCullough CJ, Burge PD: Rotary Stability of the Load-Bearing Ankle: An Experimental Study J Bone Joint Surg 62:460-464, 1980.
15. Ottosson L: Lateral Instability of the Ankle Treated by a Modified Evans Procedure. Acta Orth Scand 49:302-305, 1978.
16. Pennal GF: Subluxation of the Ankle. Can Med Assoc J 49:92-95, 1943.
17. Rubin G, Witten M: The Talar-Tilt Angle and the Fibular Collateral Ligaments: A Method for the Determination of Talar Tilt. Am J Bone & Joint Surg 42:311-326, 1960.
18. Ruth CJ: The Surgical Treatment of the Fibular Collateral Ligaments of the Ankle. Am J Bone & Joint Surg 43:229-239, 1961.
19. Sefton GK, George J, Fitton JM, McMullen H: Reconstruction of the Anterior Talofibular Ligament for the Treatment of the Unstable Ankle. Br J Bone & Joint Surg 61:352-354, 1979.
20. Storen H: A New Method for Operative Treatment of Insufficiency of the Lateral Ligaments of the Ankle Joint. Acta Chir Scand 117:501-509, 1959.
21. Watson-Jones R: Fractures and Joint Injuries, ed 4. Edinburgh, Livingstone, 1955, pp. 821-823.

CHAPTER 14

ARTHROSCOPY OF THE SUBTALAR JOINT (POSTERIOR SUBTALAR JOINT)

J. Serge Parisien, M.D.

The integrity of the subtalar joint is important for movements of inversion and eversion of the foot. Because of their complexity, conventional x-ray examination is not sufficient for their evaluation.[1]

At the present time, accurate assessment is possible through the use of some special investigative procedures, such as contrast arthrography (Figure 14-1), special x-ray projections, and CT scanning.[2-5] More recently, a direct visualization of the posterior subtalar joint by means of the arthroscope was described.[6] The availability of miniature surgical instruments has also made possible the performance of some limited surgical procedures.[7] In this chapter, we plan to review the relevant regional anatomy, the arthroscopic portals, the arthroscopic anatomy, the technique for diagnosis and surgery, and the possible indications for subtalar joint arthroscopy.

Anatomy

Three joints form the hind part of the foot: the posterior subtalar joint, the talocalcaneo-navicular joint, or anterior subtalar joint, and the calcaneocuboid joint. Two grooves placed respectively on the inferior surface of the talus and on the superior surface of the os calcis, form the tarsal canal. Its lateral opening is called the sinus tarsi. Tarsal canal and sinus tarsi divide the subtalar joints into the anterior talocalcaneo-navicular joint and posterior

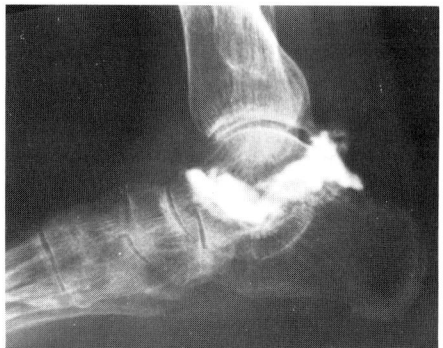

Figure 14-1. An arthrogram of the subtalar joint that shows the posterior pouch.

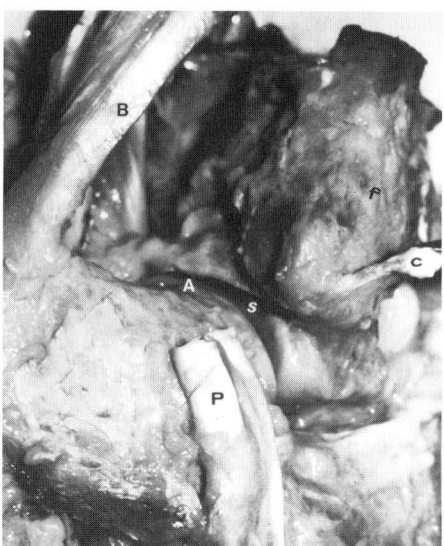

Figure 14-2. This anatomic dissection of a right foot shows (A) the posterior subtalar joint; (B) the Achilles tendon. P: Peronei, F: Fibula, c: Calcaneofibular ligament, s: Subtalar joint.

talocalcaneo joint.[8] Cahill studied the contents of the tarsal canal and found that it contains the cervical and talocalcaneo interosseous ligaments, the medial root of the inferior extensor retinaculum, a large fat pad and blood vessels. While the interosseous ligament has no role in the limitation of inversion and eversion of the subtalar joint, the cervical ligament, on the contrary, is important for the limitation of inversion.

The anterior part of the subtalar joint is a complex joint consisting of the convex head of the talus, the concave posterior part of the navicular, the anterior part of the superior surface of the os calcis, and the short plantar calcaneo-navicular ligament or "spring ligament." Posteriorly, behind the tarsal canal is located the posterior part of the subtalar joint formed by the convex superior facet of the os calcis and the concave facet of the talus. The joint line is oblique (Figures 14-2 and 14-3) and is directed upward with a convex orientation. A part of the joint is hidden by the peroneal tendon, located behind the lateral malleolous. The joint capsule has a posterior pouch and is reinforced laterally, by the talocalcaneo and the calcaneofibular ligaments. Posterior to the peroneal tendons, and superficially, the following structures are found: the small saphenous vein and the sural nerve.

Portals

Two arthroscopic portals, one anterior and one posterior to the lateral malleolus may be used for arthroscopy of the posterior subtalar joint (Figure 14-4). When a 2.2mm or a 2.7mm 10 degree arthroscope is used through the anterior portal, good visualization of the anterior aspect of the joint is provided. Visualization of the very posterior aspect of the articulation requires a posterior position of the arthroscope. With a 25 degree angle arthroscope, either portal can be used for adequate joint visualization. However, the concommitant use of the two portals is necessary, either for the use of an outflow needle or for triangulation of surgical instruments. For the use of the posterior approach, the patient must be placed in lateral decubitus position or supine, with a sand bag under the buttock. With the latter position, internal rotation of the lower limb will give sufficient exposure of the dorsolateral aspect of the foot.

Technique

Arthroscopy of the posterior subtalar joint is carried out in the operating room under spinal or general anesthesia. The patient is placed in the lateral decubitus position with the foot to be arthroscoped elevated on a bolster (Figure 14-5). The opposite lower extremity is flexed at the knee, with care being taken to avoid any abnormal pressure on the fibular head area. The supine position can also be used with a sand bag under the buttocks to allow access to the posterior lateral aspect of the foot. No leg holder is necessary, and the use of a tourniquet is optional. From the beginning of the examination, careful planning for the arthroscopic portal should be done by outlining the important landmarks. The posterior subtalar joint is a superficial structure, and the key to the anatomy is the definition of the tarsal canal and sinus tarsi. Behind these structures, the joint line is oblique and is directed upward with a convex orientation. The other important landmarks are the lateral malleolus and the peroneal tubercle. The tubercle can be palpated as a small protruberance on the lateral aspect of the os calcis between the tendons of the peroneus longus and brevis. A vertical line drawn from this tubercle passes anterior to the tip of the lateral malleolus and will cross the sinus tarsi area. No neurovascular bundle exists in this area. Posteriorly, the peroneal tendons that partially overlay the posterior part of the subtalar joint, curved around the posterior aspect of the lateral malleolus. Behind the lateral malleolus, the sural nerve is located with the small saphenous vein (Figure 14-6).

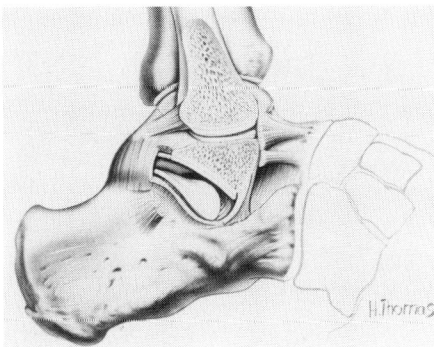

Figure 14-3. An artist's illustration of the posterior subtalar joint.

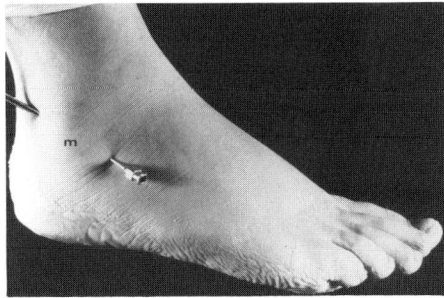

Figure 14-4. This cadaver specimen shows the position of the anterior and posterior portals with the foot in plantar flexion. m: Lateral malleolus.

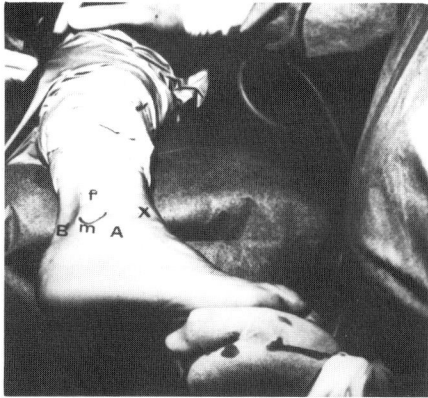

Figure 14-5. This is a patient in the lateral decubitus position. f: Fibula, B: Posterior portal, m: Tip of lateral malleolus, A: Anterior portal, x: Ankle joint.

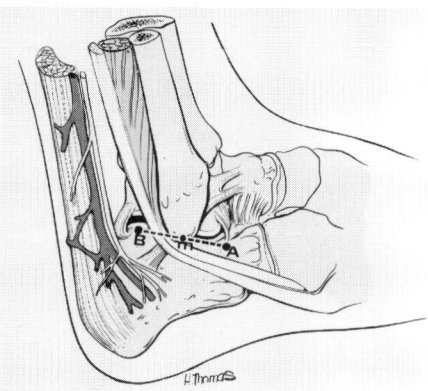

Figure 14-6. An artist's illustration of portals, with retraction of the neurovascular bundle (small saphenous vein and sural nerve). (With permission from Arthroscopy 1(1):54, 1985.)

By inverting and everting the foot, the sinus tarsi can be palpated in front of the lateral malleolus. Approximately 2cm anterior and 1cm distal to the tip of the lateral malleolus a spinal needle is placed into the joint to inflate the joint cavity with approximately 5mm to 8mm of normal saline or ringer lactate. The needle is removed and, at the same site, a small skin incision is made. An arthroscopy cannula with blunt obturator is introduced into the joint in a slightly upward direction with a firm twisting motion. The trochar is exchanged for the 2.7mm 25 degree arthroscope and the foot is held in slight inversion. If only a diagnostic arthroscopy is contemplated, the examination can be performed through an anterior portal. Joint distention is obtained with a 50cc syringe filled with normal saline or Ringer lactate, attached to the sleeve of the arthroscope by means of small plastic tubing. However, if either an outflow needle or surgical instruments are needed, a posterior portal is necessary. This portal is slightly proximal to the tip of the lateral malleolus anterior to the Achilles tendon. A too proximal placement of the portal may

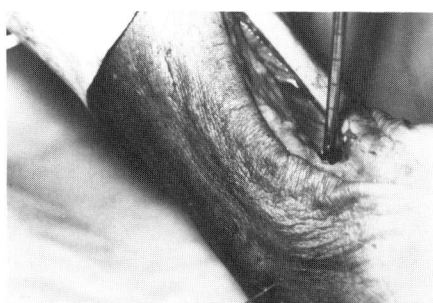

Figure 14-7. This shows the position of the arthroscope in relation to the tip of the lateral malleolus (indicated by the marker) in a left foot cadaver specimen.

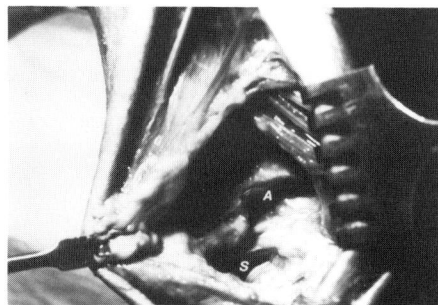

Figure 14-8. This cadaver specimen (left foot) shows the relationship of the posterior aspect of the ankle joint with the posterior subtalar joint. A: Ankle joint, S: Subtalar joint.

inadvertently enter the posterior aspect of the ankle joint (Figures 14-7 and 14-8). A spinal needle can be used posteriorly to develop a posterior portal, while the joint is being visualized through an anterior portal. The posterior portal can also be found by palpating the tip of the anteriorly placed arthroscopic obturator.

With the outflow in place, examination of the posterior subtalar joint is begun (Figure 14-9). The synovial lining of the posterior aspect of the interosseous talocalcaneo ligament is seen, then the articular cartilage of the anterior aspect of the subtalar joint is visualized, as well as the lateral aspect of the capsule and the small lateral recess of the joint. Angulation of the field of view will bring the posterior aspect of the talus and os calcis. The posterior pouch of the joint with its synovial lining can be visualized by advancing the arthroscope further posteriorly. While the scope is being maneuvered and the field of view changed, an assistant can invert and evert the foot. Even for a diagnostic arthroscopy, a switch of portal is desirable at times. Before the introduction of the arthroscope posteriorly, a small skin incision is made and a hemostat is used to move the neurovascular structures away. A disposable cannula can be used to avoid repeated penetration through the skin posteriorly. If arthroscopic surgery is required, the same two portals just outlined can be used for visualization and triangulation of surgical instruments. After completion of the procedure, the portals are closed with sutures. At times, when there is extravasation of fluid into the subcutaneous tissue, they are left open for the escape of the irrigating solution.

Postoperative Care

At the end of the procedure, a compression dressing is applied from the toes to the midcalf. The following day, this dressing is removed and ice

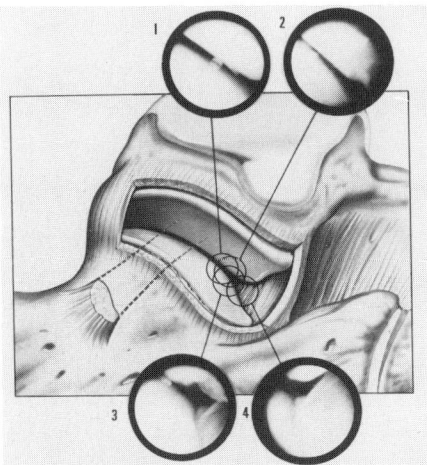

Figure 14-9. This artist's illustration shows different arthroscopic views of the anterior aspect of the posterior subtalar joint. (With permission from Arthroscopy 1(1):55, 1985.)

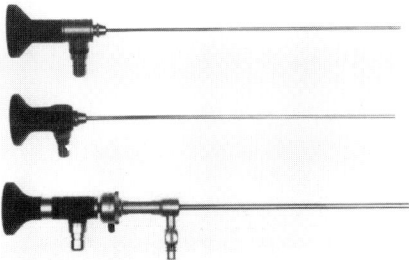

Figure 14-10. Different sizes of arthroscopes (2.2mm 10 degree, 2.7mm 10 degree, and 2.7mm 25 degree) that can be used for subtalar joint arthroscopy.

application with elevation of the leg is advised for two to three days. The patient is allowed to ambulate with the use of crutches, and weight bearing is permitted as tolerated. The sutures are removed approximately one week after the procedure, and the patient is encouraged to start range of motion exercises of the foot and ankle immediately after surgery. Once the joint swelling is completely resorbed, if indicated, the patient is referred to a physical therapist for rehabilitation under supervision.

Instrumentation

The posterior subtalar joint is a small joint and its visualization requires the use of small instrumentation. Most diagnostic arthroscopic procedures can be performed with either the 2.2mm or 2.7mm 10 degree arthroscope. We prefer the increased field of view afforded by the 2.7mm 25 degree arthroscope. A diagnostic arthroscopy can be performed by establishing only an anterior portal. Aside from the arthroscope, a spinal needle, and a 60cc syringe with small plastic tubing are needed. When surgical arthroscopy is contemplated, surgical tools, such as small grasping forceps, small motorized instruments, and disposable plastic cannula, are needed (Figures 14-10 through 14-13).

Indications

The possible indications for arthroscopic examination and surgery of the subtalar joint are:
Persistent posttraumatic symptoms.
Chondral or osteochondral fractures.
Loose bodies.
Degenerative or inflammatory arthritis.
Intraarticular adhesions.
Assessment of the status of the articular surface prior to some procedures for subtalar instability.
Patients with a history of previous injuries to the hindfoot, who continue to have pain and swelling in the subtalar joint and for whom x-rays have failed to demonstrate any abnormalities, can benefit from an arthroscopic exploration

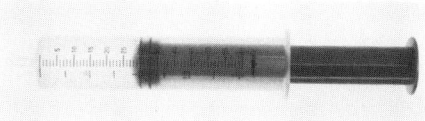

Figure 14-11. A 60cc syringe filled with normal saline.

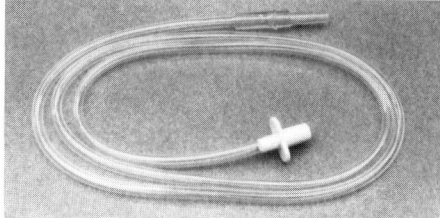

Figure 14-12. Small plastic tubing to be attached to the arthroscope sheath for irrigation during arthroscopy.

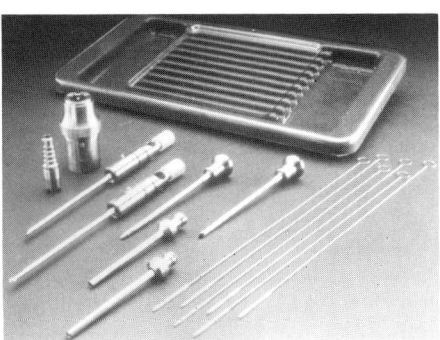

Figure 14-13. Small motorized instrumentation (Dyonics), 2.8 mm in size, with obturators, and an adapter for the cannulas and drain case.

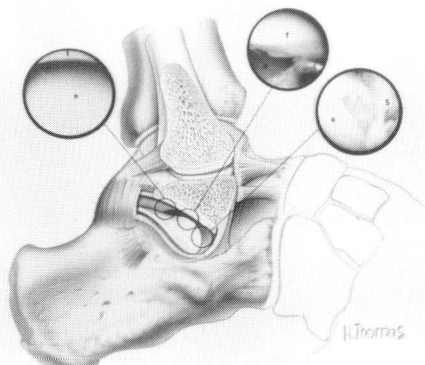

Figure 14-14. This shows the posterior subtalar joint with chondral defects and chondromalacic changes. t: Talus, o: Os calcis, s: Scar tissue.

of the joint. The presence of chondromalacia of the articular surface of chondral fracture can be ruled out. The appropriate surgical procedure, whether a chondroplasty or excision of a cartilage flap, can be performed using several triangulation techniques.

Some fractures of the os calcis or the talus can involve the articular surfaces of the posterior talocalcaneo joint. An assessment of the articular damage may be necessary at times. If loose chondral fragments are present, arthroscopic removal can be performed. In patients with suspected degenerative or inflammatory arthritis, an arthroscopic evaluation will provide more information on the condition of the articular surfaces. These patients may be helped temporarily by joint lavage. In some situations, debridement of osteophytes and hypertrophic synovium may afford temporary relief of symptoms. In suspected cases of rheumatoid arthritis, aside from the establishment of the precise diagnosis by means of direct biopsy of the synovium, the presence of chondral defect can be ascertained as well. In cases of infection of the subtalar joint, the arthroscopic technique will allow a joint debridement, followed by application of drainage tubing.

Experience has shown that in cases of arthrofibrosis of the subtalar joint, dramatic relief of pain and improvement in the range of motion can be obtained after arthroscopic excision of adhesions. While some fine adhesive bands can be broken by manipulating a small obturator through the joint, surgical instruments, such as motorized shavers or small retrograde knives, are necessary to excise thick adhesive bands. Patients with chronic instability of the subtalar joint or posttraumatic arthritis, for whom open procedures such as ligamentous reconstruction or arthrodesis are contemplated, may benefit from direct evaluation of the articular surface afforded by arthroscopy. The information obtained will help the physican decide the procedure of choice. At the same time, more information will be available for the patient regarding the type of procedure and future limitations.

Case Studies

Case 1

A 40-year-old prison guard was admitted to the hospital with pain in the subtalar joint and marked limitation of range of motion. One and on-half years prior to his admission, while trying to restrain a prisoner, he sustained an injury to his ankle. He was subsequently treated with plaster immobilization for two weeks, followed by antiinflammatory medication and physical rehabilitation. Stress x-rays failed to show any evidence of instability. Because of continued complaints of pain and instability, he was referred for arthroscopic exploration of the subtalar joint. Examination revealed marked tenderness in the sinus tarsi area and over the posterior aspect of the subtalar joint. Inversion was markedly limited. X-ray examinations were negative for fracture and osteoarthritic changes.

Under general anesthesia, the patient had an arthroscopic exploration with a 2.7 mm 25 degree arthroscope. The two portals were used for a comprehensive exploration of the joint. The articular surfaces disclosed some chondromalacic changes, and inflamed synovial tissue was also present (Figure 14-14). The motorized shaver was placed through one portal to perform a debridement of chondromalacic areas and hypertrophic synovial tissue. The portals were left open and the joint was infiltrated with 0.25% marcaine and epinephrine solution to prevent postoperative bleeding and minimize postoperative pain. A bulky dressing was applied, followed by a lighter dressing to allow ice application. The patient was started on active range of motion and ambulation with crutches the same day. He was able to discard the crutches approximately ten days following the procedure.

In two weeks, after complete healing of the wounds, an elastic support was prescribed to be worn daily. He was sent for intensive rehabilitation and placed on antiinflammatory medication for approximately two weeks. The patient was completely asymptomatic, with his range of motion much improved eight weeks after the procedure. He resumed his work three months after surgery. Because his occupation required long periods of standing, he complained for approximately two months of minimal swelling in the foot, which subsided with elevation and icing. When seen one and one-half years after the procedure, he denied any symptoms whatsoever and was very active in sports. X-rays at that time were unremarkable.

Case 2

A 32-year-old man was referred for pain in the subtalar area of his right foot. One year prior to his examination, he was treated for a bimalleolar fracture by open reduction with a cast application for two months, since the internal fixation was judged by the surgeon not to be rigid enough to allow immediate range of motion. After removal of the plaster, the patient slipped and sustained an inversion injury of the same ankle, with minimal displacement of the fracture. He was again placed in a shortleg cast for another period of two months immobilization. After removal of the cast, he was sent for intensive rehabilitation. Although he regained almost full motion of his ankle, at the end of six months of rehabilitation, his subtalar motion was

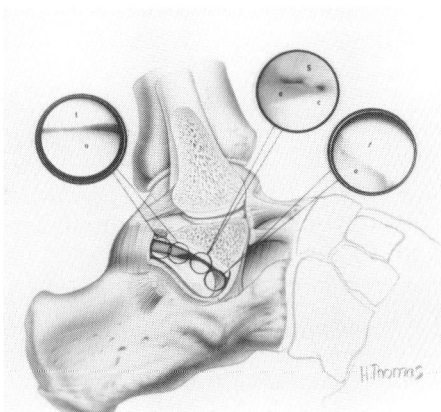

Figure 14-15. This shows the chondromalacic areas of the subtalar joint. t: Talus, o: Os calcis, c: Chondral fragment, s: Synovial reaction.

painful and limited. An arthroscopic exploration and debridement of the posterior subtalar joint (Figure 14-15) was performed at the time of the removal of the internal fixation devices. Three months after arthroscopy, the patient had a painless almost full motion of his subtalar joint, with a normal gait.

Complications

Possible complications include infection, breakage of instruments, and scuffing of the articular cartilage. Knowledge of the anatomy and proper technique will avoid injury to the neurovascular structures at risk, namely the lesser saphenous vein and the sural nerve.

Summary

Direct visualization of the posterior subtalar joint can be carried out using arthroscopic technique. With the use of small arthroscopes, ranging in size from 2.2mm to 2.7mm, much information can be obtained regarding the status of the articular cartilage and synovial lining in cases of degenerative and inflammatory arthritis. Posttraumatic pain syndrome of the hindfoot can be assessed, and limited surgical procedures such as biopsy, breakage or excision of adhesions, joint lavage, and removal of loose chondral or osteochondral bodies can be performed with less morbidity for the patient. When the technique is mastered, the foot and ankle specialist will find arthroscopy a rewarding method for the evaluation and management of some disorders of the hindfoot.

References
1. Shereff M, Johnson K: Radiographic Anatomy of the Hindfoot. Clin Orth Rel Res 177:16-22, 1983.
2. Resnick D: Radiology of the Talo-Calcaneal Articulations. Rad 3:581-586, 1974.
3. Taillard W, Meyer J, Garcia J, Blanc Y: The Sinus Tarsi Syndrome. Int Orth 5:117-30, 1981.

4. Isherwood I: A Radiographical Approach to the Subtalar Joint. Br J Bone & Joint Surg 43:566-74, 1961.
5. Smith RW, Staple TW: Computerized Tomography (CT) Scanning Technique of the Hindfoot. Clin Orth Rel Res 177:34-38, 1983.
6. Parisien JS, Vangsness T: Arthroscopy of the Subtalar Joint: An Experimental Approach. J Arth Rel Surg 1:53-57, 1985.
7. Parisien JS: Arthroscopy of the Posterior Subtalar Joint: A Preliminary Report. J Foot & Ankle, 6:219-224, 1986.
8. Cahill DR: The Anatomy and Function of the Contents of the Human Tarsal Sinus and Canal. Anat Rec 153:1-18, 1965.

CHAPTER 15

POSTOPERATIVE CARE AND PHYSICAL THERAPY

Harvey S. Kohn, M.D.
Gary N. Guten, M.D.

Arthroscopic treatment of ankles has added a new dimension to the care of our patients. The authors have developed a systematic postoperative rehabilitative regimen following ankle arthroscopy. This is tailored to the patient's individual problem and specific surgical treatment.

Following every arthroscopic procedure of the ankle, the patient is given crutches, the use of which has been arranged preoperatively. These are used until the operated ankle is relatively pain free and minimally swollen. Patients are instructed to follow the "R.I.C.E." principle of rest, ice, compression, and elevation. The authors have found that swelling following ankle arthroscopy can be a problem and is not unusual, so emphasis is placed on the use of ice and elevation for a few days following the procedure.

A postoperative posterior plaster splint has been utilized for three to five days following each surgical procedure. Later the patient is placed in a postoperative "Air Cast" splint, as necessary, for control of any residual swelling problems, once the patient begins weight bearing. Since this regimen has been instituted, postoperative pain and swelling have been noticeably diminished.

Patients are encouraged to bear weight with crutches as tolerated, except when an abrasion or drilling of an osteochondral fracture or osteochondritis dissecans is performed. In these cases, nonweight bearing is recommended for a five to six week period of time. (This has been reduced by the editor of this text to two weeks in smaller and deeper lesions.)

Each patient is given a postoperative activity program booklet in which six individual facets of the rehabilitation period are specifically spelled out. These are continually referred to and upgraded during the postoperative period. These are:
1. Activity Level.
2. Exercise.
3. Thermal Activities.
4. Support.
5. Medication.
6. Alternative Exercises.

1. Activity level begins with crutches, followed by weight bearing, as commensurate with the patient's progress and the operation performed.

2. Exercise for the ankle is encouraged with active range of motion, as soon as the postoperative splint is removed (in three to five days). Progressive resistance exercises are begun with isometrics. Isoflex exercise tubing is utilized when range of motion is full and painless. Achilles tendon stretching is encouraged with use of a towel.

3. Adjunctive thermal therapy consists of ice packs throughout the postoperative phase, especially after each prescribed exercise period. A standard ice pack or "peeled" dixie cup is utilized for ten minutes, at least three times per day. Commercial cold packs are discouraged because of the danger of thermal injury.

4. Postoperative support consists of a compression dressing with a postoperative "K Cast Splint" from the metatarsal heads to the midcalf for pain and swelling control for three to five days. This is followed by the "Air Cast" splint for weight bearing, when swelling control is required. This splint, in a smaller model, is used for returning to recreational work activities.

5. Medication, consisting of Tylenol with codeine, is given for pain control in the immediate postoperative period. Following this, the patient is encouraged to control pain with nonprescription analgesics, and, more importantly,

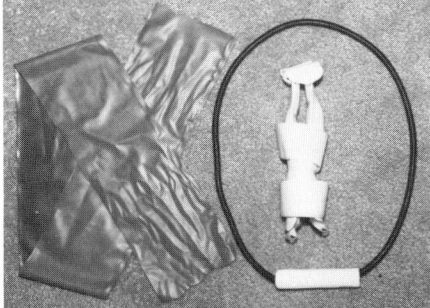

Figure 15-1. Materials used for postoperative care and physical therapy of the ankle. To the left is the theroband (blue) for ankle range of motion, stretching, and strengthening exercises. The (red) isoflex tubing at the right surrounds the air stirrup splint.

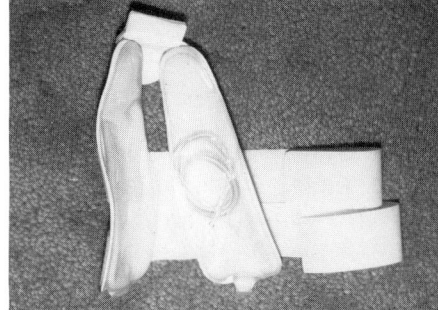

Figure 15-2. A closeup view of an air stirrup splint.

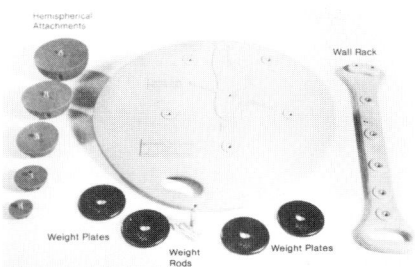

Figure 15-3. Component parts of the BAPS (Biomechanical ankle platform system) are shown.

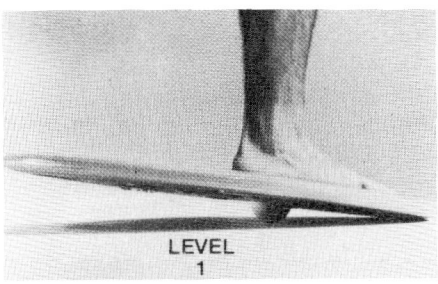

Figure 15-4. BAPS, with the patient performing plantar flexion at Level I.

modification of activities by utilization of the "R.I.C.E." principle. Sometimes an antiinflammatory medication is helpful.

6. Alternative exercises are encouraged, as soon as feasible following surgery, to encourage FESS (flexibility, endurance, speed, and strength), as well as to avoid boredom. Since many of these procedures are performed in young, active patients, used to vigorous daily activity, it is important to maintain some semblance of a fitness program. This includes biking, rowing, and swimming using a kickboard.

Exercise programs are instituted by the physical therapy department, adapted specifically to the particular arthroscopic procedures carried out:

Ankle Arthroscopic Synovectomy, Loose Body Removal, and Meniscoid Resection

A. Days 0 to 7: Crutches. Partial weight bearing as tolerated. "R.I.C.E." principle.

B. Days 0 to 7: Air splint, plus Jobst cryotherapy, if ankle is swollen. Active range of motion instruction. Towel stretch for the heel cord. Isometric exercises for the flexors and extensors of the ankle.

C. Days 14 to 21: Isoflex or Theraband tubing for plantar flexion, dorsiflexion, strengthening, and invertors/evertor exercises for the ankle, as tolerated. Continued stretching of the Achilles tendon with a towel, and wallstretching exercises. Continued active range of motion. Light biking and swimming.

D. Day 21: Above activities, plus toe raises. Increase inversion/eversion strengthening with isoflex tubing.

E. Days 28 to 42: Above exercises, plus institution of a balance training/tilt board. Cybex/Orthotron strengthening, until attaining 80% to 90% of opposite side strength. Commencement of jogging, when Cybex testing indicates that strength is 80% that of the normal ankle. Resumption of full sports activity, as tolerated, with use of the air stirrup splint, as necessary.

For arthroscopic synovectomies, swelling may occur for a longer period of time. This procedure requires crutches for several weeks, progressing to a cane in the opposite hand, until swelling is controlled and gait is normal. P.R.N. use of air stirrups.

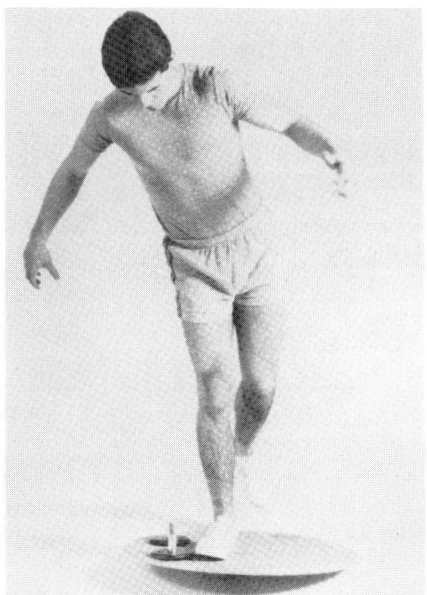

Figure 15-5. A BAPS patient performing balancing with the plate in Phase I in the anterolateral and posterolateral positions. (Courtesy R. Hawkins.)

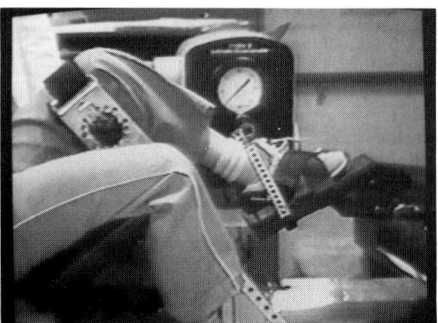

Figure 15-6. This patient is shown using the Cybex machine for passive range of motion exercises, following an abrasion arthroplasty of the ankle. This was done for an ankle with moderate, symptomatic, degenerative changes, after all forms of conservative treatment failed. (Courtesy R. Hawkins.)

Arthroscopic Abrasion or Drilling for Osteochondritis and Other Similar Lesions of the Ankle

Similar to above regimen, except for the following:

A. Days 0 to 42: Nonweight bearing on crutches for four weeks. Last two weeks toe touching (30% weight bearing) on operated side. When weight bearing with a minimal limp is demonstrated, a cane is used in the opposite hand, until normal nonpainful gait is achieved.

Exercises: No resistive exercises for six weeks post operatively. Active range of motion is emphasized on Day 7 postoperatively.

Exceptions are made for small, deep lesions. In such cases, full weight bearing can begin at two weeks. Patients who have lesions with large, shallow surface areas of the dome or the plafond that are reconstructed, abraded, and drilled should use a CPM machine for several hours, two times a day, for about a week. Then nonweight bearing should begin, as prescribed above.

Biking, and swimming begins during the third week postoperatively, using low pedal resistance, with an air stirrup splint worn on the operative ankle.

Orthotron/Cybex should begin approximately ten weeks postoperatively, as should use of the balance board.

No jogging or other running sports are permitted, until the lesion is healed. This usually takes at least six months, following an ankle abrasion or drilling procedure

CHAPTER 16

COMPLICATIONS

James F. Guhl, M.D.

There are three categories of potential complications in ankle arthroscopy. General complications, those produced by the use of general or other types of anesthesia, are well known. In addition, there are the local complications of arthroscopy of the ankle joint, just as in any joint. There are also complications of mechanical distraction, which are now to be considered in arthroscopy of the ankle. To date, in 58 cases, the author has experienced a small number of rather minor complications. A few more serious complications have been reported by others. Potential complications one must face are as follows:

Death.
Pneumonia.
Atelectasis and other cardiopulmonary complications.
Thrombophlebitis.
Pulmonary embolism.
Infections: superficial or deep.
Tourniquet, paresis, or paralysis.
Pain at the incision site.
Skin slough.
Sinus (infected sinus).
Cut or crushed nerves.
Neuroma.
Damaged vessels: hematoma, interoperative and postoperative bleeding, and hemarthrosis.
Compartment syndrome.
Scuffing of articular cartilage.
Broken instruments.
Pin cutout, pin breakage, bent pins, or pin tract infection.
Fractured malleoliis and other fractures.
Damaged ligaments, instability, tenderness, and swelling.

Damaged tendons.
Reflex sympathetic dystrophy (RSD).

Operating on the wrong joint can occur, as pointed out by Schonholtz.[1] This is inexcusable, and should be avoided by careful preoperative preparation.

One hundred and thirty-one ankle arthroscopies were performed by the author at the conclusion of the second series. Sixty-nine were performed prior to the newer methods, which were employed before November 1984, and 62 procedures were done after this date to October of 1986 (58 with distraction). Another 41 ankles were operated with distraction after the conclusion of this series and up to the time of this publication. The authors experience to date includes 172 ankle arthroscopies, 99 done with distraction. Ten of the complications described above occurred in the combined series of 131 procedures. These were quite minor in nature, except for the infected sinus tracts. The other complications listed are all potential problems, and though they did not occur, they nevertheless merit discussion when considering these new techniques.

Infection, superficial or deep, did not occur (except in the two cases of infected sinuses that will be discussed below). One portal infection occurred after the second series. There were no cases of pulmonary embolism or thrombophlebitis. This is probably due to the fact that most of the patients were young or middle-aged, and were active individuals. According to Schonholtz,[1] in order to avoid these problems, one should be aware of the past history and start aspirin three to four days postoperatively. Deaths, pneumonia, and atelectasis have not been seen.

To reduce the risk of infection the patients are asked to scrub their own extremety for 10 minutes the night before and or the morning after surgery if an arthroscope prep with Betadine gel is done at surgery. The alternative is a routine 10 minute orthopedic prep. Postoperative or intraoperative antibiotics are not routinely used.

There were two patients that had postoperative parasthesis, resulting from damage to the saphenous nerve. This caused no disability, but, nevertheless, the injuries were annoying, both to the patient and surgeon. One way of reducing this possibility is to draw the structures and the anatomical landmarks on the skin with a marking pencil prior to performing surgery.

There were no cases of damage to vessels, except for a few large veins which were tied off at the time with no longterm problems resulting. Neither postoperative arterial bleeding, hematoma formation, nor hemarthrosis has been a problem. These occurrences have been avoided in most instances, since measures were taken to prevent them. The tourniquet is released at the end of the procedure, and the joint flushed out extensively. There is enough room in the joint to cauterize any large bleeders, and, if necessary, saline may be replaced by water for this purpose.

As recommended by Schonholtz,[1] postoperative suction drains for 3 to 24 hours with one or two small tubes or drains were suggested to prevent postoperative bleeding on occasions, when indicated. Marcaine with epinephrine can be used for injection into the incisional site and for intra-articular instillation at the conclusion of surgery. To avoid hemarthrosis, aspirin should be avoided several days pre-and postoperatively, and anti-inflammatory drugs should be discontinued one week before surgery and not resumed until one week postsurgery.

Postoperative effusion can be reduced by thorough irrigation of intraarticular fragments and debris. The incisional area will also be cleansed and the occurrence of postoperative granulomas will be avoided.

Tourniquet problems were not encountered, since it was rarely left on for over one hour. If in question, it was let down, reinflated, and a check made for bleeding and compartment infiltration. Distal pulses were checked.

As far as the tourniquet is concerned, proper padding and frequent checks should be employed. There is no evidence to indicate that it is harmful in causing thrombophlebitis, in fact, it has been noted to be beneficial in preventing these problems, according to Fahmy and Patel.[2] The tourniquet was used less frequently later in the series.

The problem of sinus formation, or infected sinus, did not occur early in the first series, when the cases were mostly diagnostic. When surgery was done arthroscopically, however, later in the first series of 69, there were four cases of sinus formation. One obvious reason for this was that in triangulating, employing the accessory approaches, and when restricted to the medial or lateral side, the two incisions would be in very close proximity. Another reason is that there is very little subcutaneous tissue between the skin and joint capsule. Repeated passage of instruments added another problem. Several preventative measures were then employed, and this problem disappeared in the second series. Portal placement was kept as wide apart as possible. Plastic cannulas were used, if repeated passage of instruments was necessary. Care was taken not to engage the power in the motorized instruments, until the tips were placed in the joint under visualization. A subcutaneous stitch, or, on occasion, vertical mattress skin sutures, were utilized in closing. A short period of immobilization was often employed, from three to seven days, with crutch walking, partial, or nonweight bearing.

Two of the above four cases with sinus tracts (first series) became infected. One 17-year-old girl required immobilization with a splint, and was treated with intravenous antibiotics. She was hospitalized for one week, improved rapidly and completely, and had a good result from her surgery. The second patient developed a chronic low grade infection with pain and discomfort. This persisted for several months. The bone scan was positive. Open excision of the entire sinus was required with a secondary closure. Her result was satisfactory. She was awarded a minimal disability, since she was a compensation case.

Skin sloughs were not a problem, particularly if portals were wide apart and pressure was avoided. Also, in the elderly, local instillation of Marcaine solutions with Adrenalin into the subcutaneous portal sites was avoided, or used sparingly, since this has predisposed to skin slough (by past experience in knee surgery).

Pin breaking, bending, or cutting out was not a problem. Bending of the 3/16 inch threaded pins occurred and seemed to ensure against any ligament damage, since the pins would bend before the ligaments could stretch or tear. Larger pins are therefore not advised. Bending to some degree occurs in the

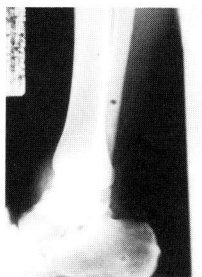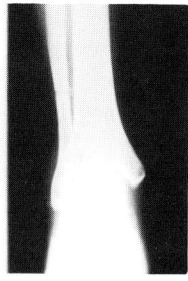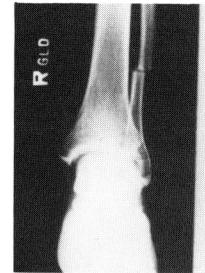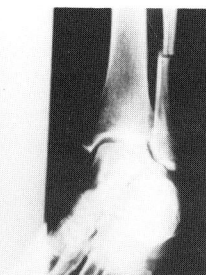

Figure 16-1. A pinhole for distraction in fibula immediately after surgery.

Figure 16-2. A fracture of the fibula at the site of the pinhole two weeks after surgery.

majority of cases. Breakage of pins occurred a few times, but was not a problem. None of the pins had to be retrieved by open surgery. The potential does exist, however, and should be kept in mind. Pins "cutting out" only occurred one time, and this was when placement was inadequate and in the fibula. The only problem was that this was not realized during the case, and therefore maximal distraction was not maintained, reducing the space for effective surgery. "Cutting out" of the distal pin did not occur to date, but this should be carefully avoided, because this could very well lead to fracture of the distal cortex of the os calcis and cause postoperative disability. This would also jeopardize the performance of surgery, as occurred in the above case.

The use of lateral x-ray for reference in pin placement is referred to in the chapter on techniques. This is especially important when pin placement is in the talus. Also, probing with a hypodermic needle should be done to be sure that the pin is placed at least ½ inch proximal to the inferior cortex of the calcaneous. These precautions need not be rigid when one has more experience. Postoperative pain or infection in the pin tract areas has not been a problem to date.

Another surgeon reported a fracture of the fibula to me, after inserting the distraction pin into that area (Figures 16-1 through 16-3). The fracture occurred several weeks after surgery. The use of the fibula, therefore, is not recommended.

Use of the talus for more direct distraction was suggested as a routine but dismissed (and is therefore not advisable) because of: a) the proximity of the neurovascular bundle, b) the danger of the pin entering the talocalcaneal joint, and c) the fact that use of the os calcis has proven to be quite adequate. The exceptions, however, as mentioned in Chapter VI, are performing an ankle arthrodesis or severe capsulitis and fibroarthrosis.

Damage to any of the ligaments of the ankle has not been observed in the second series where the new distraction method was employed. Preoperative study and previous experience with distraction of the knee would indicate that this should not be a problem. During the series, preoperative, postoperative, and intraoperative stress films substantiated this. There was no significant difference on stress x-rays, by measurement, in all cases. Also, the anterior talofibular ligament can be observed directly at surgery. There have been no postoperative complaints or signs of ligament damage even when ambulation was employed early after surgery.

The ankle joint should be distracted to only 4mm or 5mm initially. More distraction is later gained up to about 8mm during the case with ample room to do surgery. A gradual "elastic deformation" of the ligaments seems to occur, as has been noted to the medial collateral ligament in arthroscopic knee surgery.

Articular cartilage scuffing, a complication to be avoided in all arthroscopic surgery, has been reduced immensely by the distraction method. This method, and the combined use of many portals, and posterior viewing, also reduced the problem. In cases of the second series, it was kept to a bare minimum, and, in most cases, avoided completely.

Sympathetic reflex dystrophy by missed diagnosis was encountered once. Potentially, this could be one of the most annoying and, perhaps, major complications to the patient. The case referred to above did not respond to treatment by the author. The patient had continued postoperative pain and was extensively evaluated. There was no cause found other than the diagnosis of reflex sympathetic dystrophy, mostly by exclusion. Pain persisted, moderate in degree, and more annoying than disabling. The patient was then referred for consideration of a sympathetic block. There was another case of fairly obvious or clearcut malingering where relief was not obtained.

Early anterior compartment infiltration occurred in a number of cases in the first series, but was never a serious problem. Awareness and avoidance of this complication, and proper postoperative care has kept this to little more than an observation. When it does occur, secondary to excessive extravasation of saline during the procedure, the problem may be reduced by releasing the tourniquet and completing the case without delay. This occurrence subsides rapidly in the recovery room with elevation and application of warm, moist packs to the leg (ice to the ankle). It has disappeared completely after the utilization of mechanical distraction.

Broken instruments, as in any joint, are always a possibility, although a rare complication. The distraction method, better utilization of portals and sharp nonhinged or single pin specially designed instruments, should make this a very minimal threat. Should this happen, better access and visualization of the entire joint will make recovery easier by the use of a greater choice of portals and better positioning. The same precautions should be taken as with any joint: stop, think, don't panic, turn off the irrigation, and proceed cautiously. Magnetic suction devices also should be available in all operating

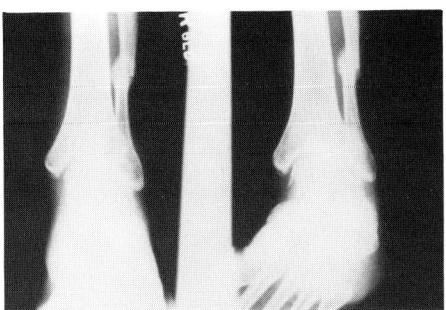

Figure 16-3. Healed fracture of the fibula.

rooms where arthroscopic surgery is performed. The use of nonmagnetic instruments should be avoided in case of breakage. This complication has not been a problem in this series.

With the use of the transmalleolar approaches, fracture of the malleolus during or after surgery was not a problem. Two or three passages of an .062 Kirschner wire were used for drilling defects of the talus. When drilling, it is important to start well above the joint line and be central in location in the malleolus, as viewed in the medial-lateral planes. The use of any one of the arthroscopic anterior cruciate ligament guides has helped a great deal in accurate transmalleolar portal placement. Transmalleolar portals should be not larger in diameter than necessary. Proper postoperative care should be employed. The channel in the bone, and especially the pin tracts as seen in x-ray, may remain visible for a long period of time after the entire area is well healed. This should be of not more concern than one or two screw holes (when fixing fractures), with subsequent removal of the screws. Of course, the use of distraction, is contraindicated in children with open epiphyses.

To date, the complications in the second series are:
2 Missed diagnoses.
2 Damaged superficial nerves.
1 Neuroma.
1 Pin cut out (fibula).
3 Painful incisional sites.

Conclusion

A final word about complications is that they can all occur, although they have been minimal in our experience. If one does, this procedure with the proper indications, follow the prescribed directions and individual equipment instructions, and has adequate experience in arthroscopic surgery, the results should should be rewarding and the complications kept at a minimum. Informal consent is always advisable. These new methods, therefore, should be safe and useful for better and more efficient surgery.

References
1.. Schonholtz GJ: Arthroscopic Surgery of the Shoulder, Elbow and Ankle. Springfield, IL, Charles C. Thomas, 1986.
2.. Patel D, Fahmy N, and Patel D: Hemostatic Changes in Post Operative Deep Vein Thrombosis Associated with the use of a Pneumatic Tourniquet. J of Bone & Joint Surgery, Vol 63A, pages 461-465, March 1981.

CHAPTER 17

ANALYSIS AND CONCLUSION

James F. Guhl, M.D.

The new techniques described above and the changes that resulted in the practice of arthroscopy and arthroscopic surgery of the ankle are analyzed and discussed in this chapter. Experience in the first series of cases, numbering 69, without the use of the mechanical distractor has been reviewed. The early procedures in that study were diagnostic for the most part. In the latter part, a total of 26 surgical procedures were performed. After the introduction of mechanical distraction, the next series numbered 62. Four of these procedures were done without distraction, two were diagnostic, and two had surgery without distraction. One of the two surgical cases without distraction was a septic ankle in a 15-year-old boy. The other case was a patient with significant instability of the ankle, which therefore did not require distraction to perform the surgery. There were 58 patients who underwent arthroscopic surgery with mechanical distraction. Two had pathology in both ankles requiring surgery. In one patient, a "second look" evaluation was done.

Of note in reviewing this experience was a learning and developmental curve, extending from the beginning of the first series well into the second, which had to be considered in the analysis of the material for preparation of this text. In order to do this in a meaningful manner, recognition of the "trial and error period" encountered must be acknowledged. The work done in the anatomy laboratory to finalize this study merits consideration. Recommendations are then presented regarding technique and surgical concepts. It is also logical that predictions regarding the future of arthroscopy of the ankle should be discussed. Table 17-1 and Figure 17-1 show the author's practice before and after the use of distraction. The surgery case performed in Figure 17-1 is shown in red. The number of diagnostic cases are in blue for the first

Table 17-1.
Diagnoses Leading to Surgery

Diagnosis	First Series	Second Series
Diagnostic	41	2
Synovial Impingement	9	29
Chronic Local Synovitis		1
Lateral Talomalleolar Joint		18
Medial Talomalleolar Joint		1
Both TM Joints		1
Posterolateral		6
Posterior (TTLF, Post Slip)		0
Meniscoid	1	2
Chronic Synovitis, General	1	1
Adhesions	1	2
Fibroarthrosis	2	2
Rheumatoid Arthritis	1	0
Synovial Chondromatosis	1	1
Infection Arthritis	0	1
Osteochondritis Dissecans (Osteochondral Fracture)	6	9
Chondral (Osteochondral Defect)		7
Dome		3
Plafond		2
Medial Malleolus		0
Lateral Malleolus		2
Loose Bodies	2	3
Osteophytes	2	2
Postfracture Pathology	1	2
Miscellaneous	1	1
TOTALS	69	62

period and in green for the second. The two series in Table 17-1 show the number of cases and the diagnoses for which surgery was performed during the twelve year span of time.

Since this is not a prospective study, the presentation of detailed results would be inappropriate, except for the limited report in Chapter IX. Furthermore, there was a necessary learning period for the development of techniques, as stated. Finally, there was not adequate time for longterm followup. However, the use of the distraction method and other techniques recently applied to ankle arthroscopy was thought to be of significant importance to merit discussion. In general, the comparison drawn by the author between the first series (before the introduction of distraction) and the second series showed that the utilization of these techniques significantly improved treatment. At followup study, these conclusions were based on answers to specific questions asked at each patient evaluation. Was the surgery successful and was the patient satisfied? What was the patient's self evaluation on a scale of one to ten? In addition, the patient was asked to compare presurgery levels of

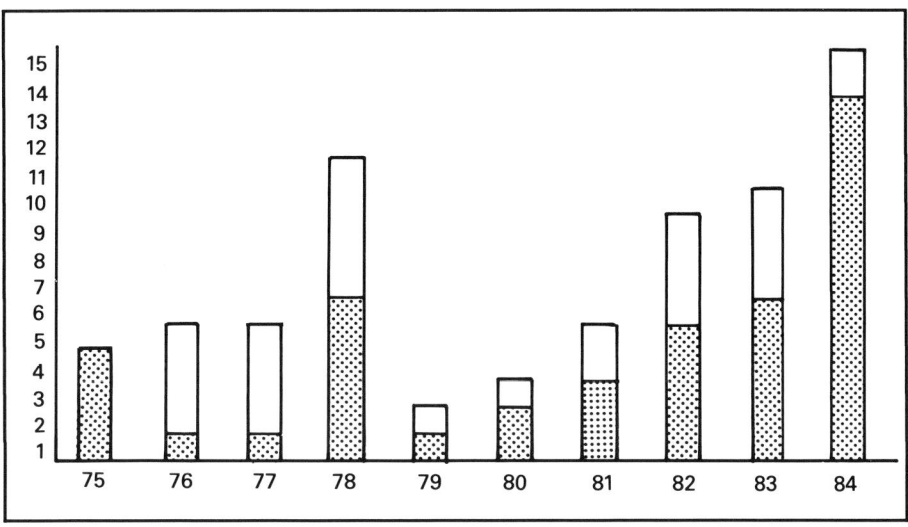

Figure 17-1. The numbers shown above represent the listing of cases done regarding diagnosis. In cases where there was more than one diagnosis, the major lesion requiring treatment was noted. The pathological diagnosis on soft tissue lesions in the first series was not subdivided, as in the second series, since the characteristics of these lesions were not fully appreciated before distraction was employed.

function and activity with postsurgery levels. Also, patient status regarding work and sports was noted. The symptoms of residual pain, swelling, locking, buckling or "instability," and clicking were taken into consideration. The findings recorded were: tenderness, swelling, limited motion (or stiffness), pain on manipulation, and, lastly, the x-ray evaluation. These facts were the basis of the author's present impressions.

In summary, as stated in Chapter IX regarding the soft tissue impingement, 26 patients of 29 were improved, and 25 were satisfied. The same conclusions could generally be drawn at this time regarding the other soft tissue lesions, osteochondritis dissecans, and other chondral and osteochondral lesions. This was demonstrated and can be noted in review of the case presentations.

To further evaluate the distraction method, pre-and postoperative stress films of 36 of the 58 patients who had undergone distraction were studied. Careful examination of 33 of these (three were lost) showed no significant difference in the pre-and postoperative angle of the ankle mortise. That is, there was no discrepancy of more than about one degree, and this was only in a few cases. There were three patients that had no preoperative x-rays, but when compared to the opposite ankle were considered within normal limits. In five of these cases, stress films were taken before and after the surgery was performed, and while the patient was still under anesthesia, with the same results. Later in the series nine cases were studied and showed no x-ray evidence of anterior-posterior instability. In summary, all findings indicated no significant increase of the ankle mortise, no clinical evidence of instability, and no further signs or symptoms of ligament damage.

Fresh or thawed frozen amputation specimens were studied to determine the amount of stress the ligaments could withstand without permanent stretching or rupture. Eight specimens were used. The pins were inserted in exactly the same manner as described for the surgical procedure. All specimens were stressed to the maximum degree, until the pins bent (in one case the distraction bar bent slightly). Four were predissected and another four were dissected to only a minimal degree to observe the difference in the angle of the ankle mortise. In two specimens the ankles were kept distracted for over 45 minutes. There was no clinical evidence on final examination of these specimens to suggest any increase in the ankle mortise or stretching or tearing of the ligaments.

The maximum time the ankle was held in distraction during surgery was a little under one hour and many of these were less. The greatest average distraction measurement was 7mm to 8mm of increased distance of the talus from the tibia, mostly on the lateral side. In many cases, distraction was carried out until bending of the 3/16 threaded Steinman pin occurred.

Experience noted in the second series with application of these techniques led to continued improvement in the performance of ankle arthroscopy. A significant degree of knowledge was experienced regarding arthroscopy of this joint, methods of treatment, and pathology.

In 90% of the ankles arthroscoped, distraction proved to be of great help to obtain the best advantage in performing surgery. This was true, even if there was initial minimal instability. With moderate instability (as in a few cases) distraction was not necessary to adequately visualize and explore the pathology. In most instances, however, it was found best for maintenance of the interarticular space of the ankle to comfortably and safely perform surgery.

With the utilization of this method, 90% of the cases were fairly easy from the standpoint of application of technique. Even after some experience was gained, the remainder were somewhat difficult. This was mostly in obtaining entry into these joints, either because of tight ligaments or, more often, because of obstruction from chronically inflamed synovial tissue. It was necessary to establish adequate visualization, in some cases, by performing an extensive debridement after maximum distraction was obtained. Also, in cases of degenerative arthritis, capsulitis, and fibroarthrosis, evaluation and treatment were more challenging.

The ankleholder proved to be a significant aid, placing the ankle firmly in the optimum controlled position for complete and adequate exposure, along with distraction and utilization of all approaches.

The majority of arthroscopic surgery in the ankle joint can be done by triangulation, utilizing the anterior approaches. The posterolateral portal, therefore, appeared necessary in only a limited number of cases. In several cases of loose bodies located posteriorly, and in many instances of chondral pathology, it proved to be invaluable. Application of this approach may increase with further knowledge of pathology in the posterior compartment. In order to perform a complete diagnostic examination of the patient's ankle joint, the posterolateral portal will be more frequently required. This format should be found to be the same, to some degree, as was the need for the use of the posterior approaches in the knee, as time passed, to perform a comprehensive examination.

More pathology was found than was expected in the second series. There were chondral defects of the tibial plafond, synovial impingement lesions in the posterolateral aspect of the joint, and certain treatable lesions in the arthritic ankle. The percentage of pathology found and treated was quite high. This was the result of extensive preoperative preparation, clinical evaluation, and choice of x-ray diagnostic procedures. There were very few negative examinations or purely diagnostic cases (about 5%). This incidence was less than with arthroscopy of the knee and shoulder, as noted by the author in his experience and in noting the experience of other arthroscopic surgeons.

The overall results that can be expected from arthroscopic surgery of the ankle with these techniques appears to be much improved over that in the past. This was brought out by a general comparison of the second series to the first. In the earlier study, patients in some cases continued to have symptoms but nothing was found. It is obvious in retrospect, that a good number of pathological entities could be and were missed. Also, lesions were found in patients in the second series that were missed on previous arthroscopic examination either by the author or in several cases by the referring orthopedic surgeon where distraction was not used. This has been illustrated by several examples in this text. A number of immediate results of arthroscopic surgery of the ankles were quite surprizing and dramatic when these techniques were employed. There was in most cases significant relief of pain from excision of the synovial impingement tissue, particularly in those lesions in the posterolateral corner of the ankle joint. This was true when these entities appeared to be quite small in size and not initially thought to be significant.

No major complications (but a few minor ones) occurred in the 58 cases, in which distraction was employed. A few significant problems were reported to the author by other orthopedic surgeons. This technique, therefore, appears to be safe, based on the experience in the second series and the laboratory experiments.

The development of four sinus tracts (two infected) in the first series has been eliminated in the second by improving the technique. Also, a reduced incidence of swelling about the ankle has been noted. Fewer instances of infiltration into the compartments of the leg, less scuffing, and greater ease in performing surgery were demonstrated. The latter has now become far less demanding.

Operative time, in most cases, should now be 40 minutes or less. In the author's second series, there was additional time needed to develop new techniques by the "trial and error" method. There was also further delay in performing surgery because of the need to utilize 35mm and video documentation, from both inside and outside. Stress x-rays were also used on occasion. All of these were necessary for the preparation of formal presentations and for the material in this text.

The Future

It is expected that posterior triangulation and the use of transmalleolar approaches will continue to be refined and developed, and that the results will be further improved. Longterm followup studies and "second looks," especially in osteochondral lesions, will yield more knowledge regarding indications, techniques, postoperative care, and rehabilitation. More case studies will clarify the techniques and indications for performing successful ankle arthrodesis arthroscopically, and for doing corrective surgery of the unstable ankle. Pathology and anatomy encountered in arthroscopy of the posterior ankle joint, as well as the subtalar joint, will be better correlated with experience. Lesions such as the "meniscus" of the ankle, as described by Hamilton,[1] or th pathological transverse tibiofibular ligament, or posterior slip, as described by Chen[2] and Ikeuchi[3] will be more thoroughly understood. Better correlation with x-ray procedures should occur and make the choice of these more practical.

The application of these methods in sports medicine injuries will be established. The indications, contraindications, and the development of arthroscopic surgery in arthritis of the ankle will be further clarified. Finally, various questions should be presented and serve as the stimulus for future scientific papers regarding arthroscopic surgery of this joint.

References
1. Hamilton H: Personal Communication, 1986.
2. Chen Y: Arthroscopy of the Ankle Joint. In: Watanabe M: Arthroscopy of Small Joints. New York, Igaku-Shoin, 1985.
3. Ikeuchi H: Personal Communication, 1987.

Index

Adhesions, 82-83, 90-91, I Fig. 9-3
Aiming device, 44
Analysis of ankle arthroscopy,
 153-158; *see also* Ankle arthroscopy
Anatomy, 7-12
 arthroscopic, 13-23
 bones in, 9
 ligaments in, 10-12
 of posterior subtalar joint, 133-134
 surface, 7-9
 talus in, 9-10
Andrew's technique, 60-61
Ankle arthroscopy
 analysis of, 153-158
 anatomy in, 7-12
  arthroscopic, 13-23
 in chondral and osteochondral
  lesions, 107-117
 in chronic lateral ankle instability,
  123-131
 complications of, 147-152
 differential diagnosis and, 69-78
 future of, 158
 history of, 1-6
 indications and contraindications for,
  64-67
 instrumentation in, 37-48
 in osteochondritis dissecans, 95-106
  physical therapy and, 143-146
  portals and techniques in, 49-62;
   see also Techniques
  posterior subtalar joint and,
   133-142
  postoperative care and, 143-146
  radiological techniques and, 25-36
  in synovial pathology, 79-94; *see
   also* Synovitis
  tibiotalar arthrodesis in, 119-122
Ankle holder, 44, 45
Ankle instability repair, 123-131; *see
 also* Lateral ankle instability repair
Ankle pain, diseases causing, 70-74
Anterior impingement lesions, 111-112
Anterior periarticular ankle problems,
 75-76
Anterocentral approach, 55, 56-57
Anterolateral approach, 55-56
Anteromedial portal, 55, 57-58

Arthritis, 65
 degenerative, 112-114, 116-117, I
  Fig. 11-32 through 11-38
 gouty, 81
 rheumatoid, 80, I Fig. 9-1, 9-2
 traumatic, 112-114
Arthrodesis, arthroscopic tibiotalar,
 119-122
Arthrography, 31-33
Arthroscope, 38-39
Arthroscopic abrasion, postoperative
 care and, 146
Arthroscopic anatomy, 13-23
Arthroscopic cannulas, disposable, 40
Arthroscopic tibiotalar arthrodesis,
 119-122
 contraindications to, 122
 indications for, 121
 operative technique for, 119-121
Arthroscopy pump, 45, 47

Basket forceps, 41
Biomechanics of chronic lateral ankle
 instability, 124-125
Bones, 9

Cameras, video, 39
Cannulas, disposable arthroscopic, 40
Chondral and osteochondral lesions,
 64-65, 107-117
 arthritis and, 114-117, I Fig. 11-1
  through 11-52
 case reviews and, 114-117, I Fig. 11-1
  through 11-52
 fractures and, 114, I Fig. 11-39
  through 11-52
 loose bodies and, 110-111, 115, I
  Fig. 11-6 through 11-21
 osteophytes and, 111-112, I Fig.
  11-22 through 11-31
 plafond lesions and, 109-110,
  114-115, I Fig. 11-4, 11-5
 synovial impingement syndrome
  and, 84-85, 89, I Fig. 9-5
  through 9-11, 9-21, 9-22
 talar dome defects and, 108-109, I
  Fig. 11-1 through 11-3

Chondromatosis, synovial, 80-81, 91, I
  Fig. 9-26 through 9-30
Classification
  of synovitis, 79-80
Complications, 147-152
  of posterior subtalar joint
    arthroscopy, 141
Computed tomography, 33-34
Contraindications for arthroscopy,
    66-67
  and tibiotalar arthrodesis, 122
Conventional radiography, 26-27
Conventional tomography, 30-31
Crohn's disease, 81
Curettes, 41, 42
Cutting instruments, 41

Degenerative arthritis, 112-114,
    116-117, I Fig. 11-32 through 11-38
Differential diagnosis, ankle problems
    and, 69-78
  functional, 75
  intraarticular, 77
  periarticular, 75-77
  systemic, 69-75
Disease
  ankle pain and, 70-74
  Crohn's, 81
Disposable arthroscopic cannulas, 40
Distraction, mechanical, 44-45, 46,
    52-53
Drilling for osteochondritis dessicans,
    98
  postoperative care and, 146

Etiology of osteochondritis dissecans,
    95-96
Excisional instruments, 40-43

Forceps
  basket, 41
  grasping, 42
  pituitary, 42
Fractures, 114, 117, I Fig. 11-39
  through 11-52
Functional ankle problems, 75

Ganglion, 89-90, I Fig. 9-23
Gas arthroscopy, 47

Gouty arthritis, 81
Grasping forceps, 42

Hand instruments, 40-42
History of arthroscopy, 1-6
Holder, ankle, 44, 45

Idiopathic periarticular ankle
    problems, 77
Impingement lesions
  anterior, 111-112
  posterior, 87-88, I Fig. 9-16
    through 9-20
  posterolateral, 85, 89-90, I Fig. 9-12
    through 9-14, 9-23
  synovial, 84-85, 89, I Fig. 9-5
    through 9-11, 9-21, 9-22
  posterior, 87-88, 112, I Fig. 9-16
    through 9-20
Incidence of osteochondritis
    dissecans, 96
Indications for arthroscopy, 64-66
  for posterior subtalar joint, 138-139
  and tibiotalar arthrodesis, 121
Infectious synovitis, 88, 91-92, I Fig.
    9-31 through 9-34
Inflow systems, 39
Instability, repair of, 123-131; *see also*
    Lateral ankle instability repair
Instrumentation, 37-48
  accessory, 44-47
  excisional, 40-43
  posterior subtalar joint arthroscopy
    and, 137, 138, 139
  for repair, 43, 44
  retrieving, 44, 45
  for viewing, 38-40
Insufflator for arthroscopy in gas
    medium, 47
Intraarticular ankle problems, 77
Intra-articular shaver system, 42-43,
    44

Lateral ankle instability repair, 123-131
  arthroscopic technique in, 125-127
  biomechanics in, 124-125
  case report of, 129-130
  clinical problem and, 123-124
  complications of, 128
  results of, 127

Lateral periarticular ankle problems, 76-77
Lesions, chondral and osteochondral, 107-117; *see also* Chondral and osteochondral lesions
Ligaments, 10-12
Light cables, 38-39
Local synovitis, 80, 83-89, I Fig. 9-4 through 9-20
Location osteochondritis dissecans and, 96
Loose bodies, 110-111, 115, I Fig. 11-6 through 11-21
 postoperative care and, 145

Magnetic resonance imaging, 34-36
Malleolar osteotomy, 98
Mechanical distraction, 44-45, 46, 52-53
Medial periarticular ankle problems, 76
Meniscoid, 85-86, I Fig. 9-15
 postoperative care and, 145
Motion-record studies, 36
Motorized instrumentation, 42-43, 44

Needles, spinal, 40
Nodule, 89-90, I Fig. 9-23
Nonspecific synovitis, 80, 82-83, I Fig. 9-3

Operating room setup, 50-52
Osteochondral lesions, 64-65, 107-117; *see also* Chondral and osteochondral lesions
Osteochondritis dissecans, 95-106, I Fig. 10-1 through 10-41
 analysis of, 102-104
 case reviews of, 100-102, I Fig. 10-5 through 10-28
 conservative versus surgical treatment of, 97
 drilling of base and, 98
 etiology of, 95-96
 incidence of, 96
 location of, 96, I Fig. 10-1
 malleolar osteotomy and, 98
 mechanism of injury in, 96
 postoperative care and, 98-99, 146
 stages of, 97
 structural characteristics of, 96-97
 treatment results and, 99-100
 x-rays and, 99
Osteophytes, 111-112, 115-116, I Fig. 11-22 through 11-31
Osteotomy, malleolar, 98

Pain, diseases causing, 70-74
Parisien technique, 61-62
Periarticular ankle problems, 75-77
Physical therapy, 143-146
Pigmented villonodular synovitis, 81
Pituitary forceps, 42
Plafond lesions, 109-110, 114-115, I Fig. 11-4, 11-5
Portals, 49-62; *see also* Techniques
 anteromedial, 55, 57-58
 posterior subtalar joint and, 134-135
Positioning, 50-52
Posterior impingement lesions, 87-88, 112, I Fig. 9-16 through 9-20

Synovitis
 case reviews in, 88-92
 classification of, 79-80
 infectious, 88, 91-92, I Fig. 9-31 through 9-34
 local, 80, 83-89, I Fig. 9-4 through 9-20
 nonspecific, 80, 82-83, I Fig. 9-3
 specific, 79-81, I Fig. 9-1 through 9-3
Systemic ankle problems, 69-75

Talar dome defects, 108-109, I Fig. 11-1 through 11-3
Talus, 9-10
Techniques, 49-62
 alternate, 60-62
 anterocentral approach and, 55, 56-57
 anterolateral approach and, 55-56
 anteromedial portal and, 55, 57-58
 for arthroscopy, 53-54
 in tibiotalar arthrodesis, 119-121
 for chronic lateral ankle instability stapling repair, 123-131
 mechanical distraction and, 52-53
 operating room setup in, 50-52

Posterior subtalar joint arthroscopy, 133-142
   anatomy in, 133-134
   case studies in, 140-141
   complications of, 141
   indications for, 138-139
   instrumentation for, 137, 138, 139
   portals for, 134-135
   postoperative care and, 137-138
   technique for, 135-137
Posterior-lateral periarticular ankle problems, 76
Posterior-medial periarticular ankle problems, 76
Posterolateral approach, 57, 58, 59
Posterolateral lesion, 85, 89-90, I Fig. 9-12 through 9-14, 9-23
Postoperative care, 143-146
   osteochondritis dissecans and, 98-99
   for posterior subtalar joint arthroscopy, 137-138
Probes, 40, 41
Pump, arthroscopy, 45, 47

Radioisotope scanning, 28-30
Radiological techniques, 25-36
   in arthrography, 31-33
   in computed tomography, 33-34
   in conventional radiography, 26-27
   in conventional tomography, 30-31
   in magnetic resonance imaging, 34-36
   in motion-record studies, 36
   in radioisotope scanning, 28-30
   in stress x-rays, 27-28
   in xeroradiography, 36
Rasps, 41, 42
Repair instrumentation, 43, 44
Retrieving instruments, 44, 45
Rheumatoid arthritis, 80, I Fig. 9-1, 92

Scanning, radioisotope, 28-30
Scissors, 41
Shaver system, intra-articular, 42-43, 44
Soft tissue impingement, posterior, 87-88, I Fig. 9-16 through 9-20
Soft tissue pathology, 64, 79-94; see also Synovitis
Specific synovitis, 80, 79-81, I Fig. 9-1 through 9-3
Spinal needles, 40
Stapling for chronic lateral ankle instability, 123-131; see also Lateral ankle instability repair
Stress x-rays, 27-28
Subtalar joint arthroscopy, posterior; see Posterior subtalar joint arthroscopy
Synovectomy, postoperative care and, 145
Synovial chondromatosis, chronic, 80-81, 91, I Fig. 9-26 through 9-30
Synovial impingement syndrome, 84-85, 89, I Fig. 9-5 through 9-11, 9-21, 9-22
   portals and, 54-55
   positioning in, 50-52
   for posterior subtalar joint arthroscopy, 135-137
   posterolateral approach and, 57, 58, 59
   trans-achilles tendon approach and, 58
   transmalleolar approaches and, 58-60
Tibiotalar arthrodesis, arthroscopic, 119-122
Tomography, 30-31
Trans-achilles tendon approach, 58
Transmalleolar approaches, 58-60
Trauma
   arthritis and, 112-114
   osteochondritis dissecans and, 96

Video cameras, 39
Viewing instruments, 38-40
Villonodular synovitis, pigmented, 81

Xeroradiography, 36
X-rays, 26-27
   stress, 27-28

NO LONGER THE PROPERTY
OF THE
UNIVERSITY OF R.I. LIBRARY